INTERMITTENT FASTING COOKBOOK

Publications International, Ltd.

Photographs and art on front cover and pages 49 and 113 copyright © Shutterstock.com.

Pictured on the front cover *(top to bottom):* Chicken and Quinoa Bowl *(page 48)* and Rotini Pasta Salad with Chicken *(page 112).*

Pictured on the back cover *(clockwise from top left):* Spinach Veggie Wraps *(page 52),* Spicy Chicken Rigatoni *(page 116),* Texas Caviar *(page 178)* and Spatchcock Chicken and Vegetables *(page 140).*

Contributing Writer: Lisa Brooks

ISBN: 978-1-63938-048-0

Manufactured in China.

8 7 6 5 4 3 2 1

Microwave Cooking: Microwave ovens vary in wattage. Use the cooking times as guidelines and check for doneness before adding more time.

Note: This publication is only intended to provide general information. The information is specifically not intended to be a substitute for medical diagnosis or treatment by your physician or other health care professional. You should always consult your own physician or other health care professionals about any medical questions, diagnosis, or treatment. (Products vary among manufacturers. Please check labels carefully to confirm nutritional values.)

Let's get social!
⊙ @Publications_International
⨍ @PublicationsInternational
www.pilbooks.com

CONTENTS

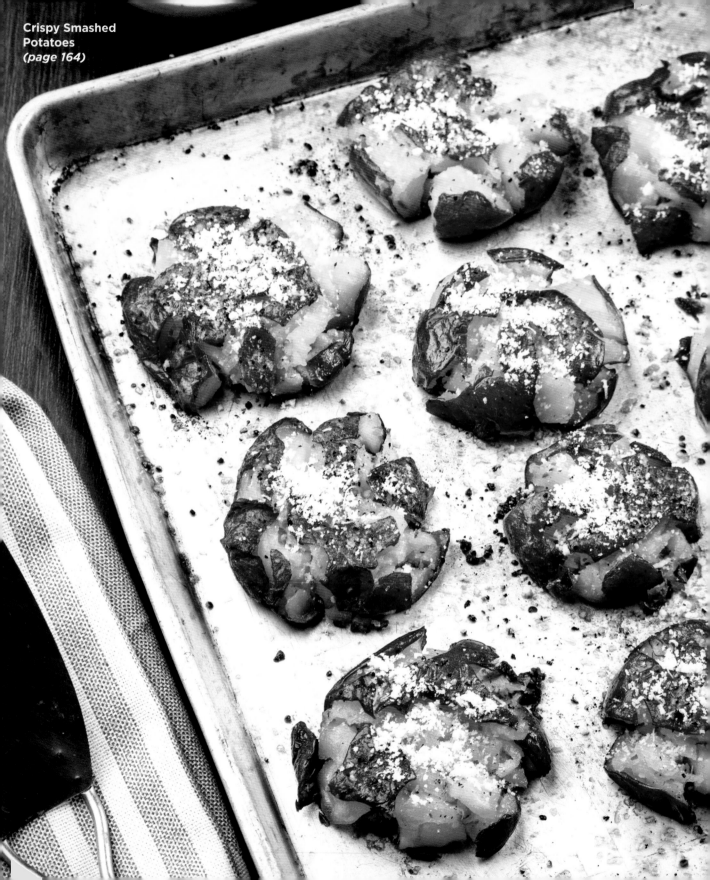

Crispy Smashed
Potatoes
(page 164)

INTRODUCTION

Food for Thought

If you were to ask a random group of people for their New Year's resolutions, chances are many of them would say the same things: lose a bit of weight, gain more energy, eat healthier foods. In fact, most of us could benefit from exercise and healthy eating, especially considering that an astounding two thirds of Americans are overweight or obese.

Often, when we resolve to live a healthier lifestyle, our first inclination is to hit the gym. Exercise certainly results in plenty of benefits, including lowering blood pressure, preventing heart disease, and boosting mood. But recent studies have shown that exercise has a much less profound effect on weight loss than we previously believed. It can be discouraging to spend hours at the gym, only to see no difference in the scale or in the way our clothes fit. So what does work? Experts say that the most significant changes occur when we pay more attention to our eating habits.

What you eat – and how you eat – have a much bigger impact on weight and health than exercise alone. A quick perusal of social media provides a look into the wide array of diets, eating plans, and recipes that are getting all the buzz right now. Popular diets come and go, some gaining large followings

of adherents while others fizzle out and are lost to the past. But even the trendiest of these diets can be customized to fit into a method of eating that has not only gained a large following of devotees who swear by its effectiveness, but has also been used by health advocates for centuries: intermittent fasting.

Fasting has been practiced since ancient times for religious and cultural purposes, and also for therapeutical and medical purposes. Records of the practice go back to at least the 5th century B.C., when the famous Greek physician Hippocrates, who is often called the "Father of Medicine," prescribed fasting to his patients. Hippocrates believed that abstaining from food, and sometimes even water, helped the body heal itself from a variety of maladies. Whether he was correct or not, most of us don't want to completely cut food and water out of our daily nutritional intake. But fasting intermittently is an attainable goal for many people.

The Whats, Hows, and Whys

It may be surprising to learn that all of us, whether we realize it or not, fast to a certain extent. That's exactly what you're doing when you sleep at night! The word "breakfast" literally means "breaking the fast," and most of us "fast" for at least seven to nine hours at a time before tucking into our morning bacon and eggs. For humans, this occasional fasting is actually quite natural. Thousands of years ago, when our ancestors had to hunt and gather their food, fasting was often necessary simply because food was not always available. Because of this, our bodies evolved to withstand long periods without nourishment.

Fortunately, in modern times we need to hunt no further than the grocery store to find our food. But that doesn't mean that we can't still benefit from an occasional fast. And even though fasting requires abstaining from food for a period of time, let's be clear: intermittent fasting is not a "starvation diet"! Practitioners of this way of eating consider it a method that can safely be incorporated into a healthy lifestyle. Like the naturally occurring overnight fast that most of us practice, intermittent fasting is an eating plan that cycles between periods of fasting and eating. And in a world where food is readily available, sedentary lifestyles are common, and illnesses like diabetes and heart disease are rampant, this type of eating plan can be greatly beneficial.

There are several different ways to follow intermittent fasting, but they all operate with the same concept: a fixed, alternating schedule of eating and fasting. No matter which schedule you choose to follow, all intermittent fasting works the same way. Usually, when we're eating three meals a day (plus snacks!) our bodies use whatever food was last eaten to provide us with energy. But by delaying the time between meals,

the body burns through its sugar stores and begins to burn fat. This is a process known as metabolic switching, and it has been shown to not only facilitate weight loss, but also to improve the function of the brain and to prevent metabolic and cardiovascular disease.

Metabolic switching isn't the only process that occurs during intermittent fasting. The practice has been shown to lower blood sugar levels and raise levels of human growth hormone, or HGH, which is an essential component of muscle gain and fat loss. Intermittent fasting also helps to initiate a process called "autophagy," which is the body's way of removing damaged or unnecessary cells. Malfunctions in this process have been linked to diseases including Alzheimer's disease and cancer, so it is important that the body be able to effectively engage in autophagy. Some studies have shown that intermittent fasting is so good at aiding autophagy that laboratory animals who are fed in this way not only live longer, but also age more slowly than their counterparts.

The many benefits of intermittent fasting make it an appealing option for anyone who wants to lose weight, lower blood pressure, prevent type 2 diabetes and heart disease, and protect against neurodegenerative disorders.

Make a Plan

Like any diet or eating plan, intermittent fasting is not for everyone. But if you're up for the challenge – and have clearance from your doctor – the first step is to choose a schedule that works best for you. It's important to stick to a set timetable, so you can plan your meals around the days and hours of your fast.

The most popular intermittent fasting plan is called the 16:8 method. This simply means that during the course of a 24-hour day, you fast for 16 hours and only eat during the remaining eight hours. Many fasters especially like this plan since the majority of the fasting hours are taken up by sleeping, and there are no restrictions on the amount of calories that can be eaten during the eight-hour eating window. A simple way to stick to this plan would be to skip breakfast, then eat a normal lunch and dinner between noon and 8 p.m. Some people stick to this schedule seven days a week, whereas others choose two or three days a week to be fasting days.

If 16 hours of fasting is too much, another option is the 14:10 method. As its name suggests, this plan requires only 14 hours of fasting, with a 10-hour eating window. This plan allows for a more "normal" eating schedule, with many people opting to begin fasting by 7 or 8 p.m. The 10-hour meal period provides plenty of time for a reasonable breakfast, lunch, and dinner, while cutting out the late-night snacks that trip up so many of us.

The 5:2 method is another popular intermittent fasting plan. While the 16:8 and 14:10 methods only restrict the hours in which meals are eaten, the 5:2 method restricts calories on two days of the week. Those who choose this plan eat normally five days a week, but eat only 400 to 500 calories (approximately 25 percent of normal calorie intake) on two non-consecutive days of the week.

Each of these plans is simple to follow for most people, with easily attainable goals. But for those who are interested in taking the "fasting" part of intermittent fasting more seriously, alternate day fasting is an option. With this plan, fasting lasts for 24 hours. So, if you finish dinner at 8 p.m. on Monday, your next meal won't be until 8 p.m. on Tuesday. You can then eat normally for 24 hours, and then repeat the cycle. If fasting altogether is too difficult, the plan can be modified to include up to 500 calories on fasting days.

In for the Long (or Short) Haul

When embarking on an intermittent fasting journey, you may wonder how long to continue sticking to your new eating plan. The answer depends on your objectives and on how easily you are able to incorporate your fasting plan into your lifestyle. Some people fast for only a few weeks or months, whereas others make a lifetime commitment to this type of eating plan. Because it is such a flexible eating method, there are no set "rules" when it comes to the length of an intermittent fasting program.

But when it comes to reaching your goals, a fasting program may only be necessary for a short time. For instance, if your goal is weight loss, you may begin to see changes within as little as two weeks of starting an intermittent fasting program. You can then continue with the fasting plan until you've reached your goal weight, however long it takes. But if your goal is to reverse insulin resistance, it could take significantly longer to see changes. You may need to fast for six months or longer to reap the blood-sugar-lowering benefits of this eating method. And no matter what your goal is, adding an exercise plan to your schedule will help to accelerate results.

If you do decide to end a fasting program, you may want to consider incorporating a "maintenance" fasting plan into your lifestyle. Many experts recommend such a plan after an intermittent fasting program, otherwise there is a risk of negating all the benefits achieved with the diet. If you lose ten pounds with intermittent fasting, but go right back to your old eating habits once you hit your goal, those ten pounds could come right back. It would be a shame to lose the results of all that hard work!

With a maintenance fasting plan, intermittent fasting is still a part of your lifestyle, but perhaps not as often. Instead of using the 16:8 or 14:10 methods every day of the week, they can be used a few days a week. The 5:2 or alternate day fasting methods could be cut down to one day a week. Or, instead of cutting down the days of a fast, an "on/off" approach can be used. This is where you follow an intermittent fasting plan for a set amount of time, then return to your regular way of eating for the same amount of time, and then continue to alternate this schedule. For example, you can fast for a month, eat regularly for a month, and then repeat the cycle over and over. You can also choose any length of time you want – fast on/off for two weeks, two months, etc. – but the key is to be consistent.

Clean vs. Dirty

It should be noted that with any fasting plan, certain liquids are always permitted and encouraged during fasting periods. It's important to stay hydrated during a fast, so drinking plenty of water is essential. But water isn't the only thirst-quenching option you can consume during a fast. What you choose to drink can depend on how "clean" or "dirty" you want your fast to be.

A "clean" fast is a fast in which only water or non-caloric beverages are consumed for the duration of the fast. Water, sparkling water, unsweetened tea, and black coffee are all great choices. Some fasting "purists" claim that beverages like coffee are still not "clean" enough, since a cup can contain around five calories and negligible amounts of carbohydrates and minerals. But these miniscule amounts of calories and carbohydrates are not enough to counteract the benefits of a fasted state, so go ahead and enjoy a cup!

In contrast, a "dirty" fast allows a small amount of calories during a fast, usually between 50 and 100. This means you could add some creamer or sweetener to your coffee or tea, including cream, milk, honey, or maple syrup. Or, jazz up your water with some lemon or lime juice. You could even drink a cup of low-calorie chicken or vegetable broth, for something a bit more "meal"-like. Just be sure to keep a careful log of what you ingest, as the calories can add up quickly. For example, if you add just one tablespoon of cream to your coffee, you've already reached more than 50 calories.

Dirty fasting also allows artificial sweeteners, but be cautious: some of these can cause an increase in appetite—definitely an unwanted side-effect during a fast—so you may have to experiment with different types of sweeteners to find one that works best.

Choosing to go with clean or dirty fasting is really just a matter of preference. It's unlikely that the small amount of calories, carbohydrates, and fat consumed during a dirty fast could hinder your progress, but if you're not seeing results using a dirty fast, you can always switch to clean fasting to see if it provides the extra boost you need. But many fasters find that the calories consumed during dirty fasting provide enough satiety to help them stick with a fasting program longer. In fact, if you find yourself unable to stick to a fast long enough to see results while you're clean fasting, switching to dirty fasting may ultimately help you fast longer and see more progress. You can also alternate the two techniques for the length of your fast.

What exactly can you consume during clean and dirty fasting?

FOR CLEAN FASTING, ZERO-CALORIE OPTIONS INCLUDE:

water

unflavored sparkling water

unsweetened tea

black coffee

DIRTY FASTING OPTIONS INCLUDE:

1 tbsp cream (51 calories)

1 tbsp whole milk (9 calories)

1 tbsp unsweetened almond milk (2 calories)

1 tsp honey (21 calories)

1 tsp maple syrup (17 calories)

1 cup chicken broth (40 calories)

Water plus the juice of one lemon or lime (12 calories)

Artificially sweetened drinks

Fasting Flexibility

No matter what or how you eat, any positive or negative effects of your diet will come about through consistency. If you consistently eat a poor diet, it can result in weight gain, a lack of energy, or even a risk for deadly diseases. Conversely, if you consistently eat a healthy diet, it can result in weight loss, an abundance of energy, and a lowered risk of disease. However, sticking with any healthy eating program is sometimes easier said than done. After all, life is always presenting us with challenges and throwing curveballs, and falling back into old unhealthy habits can be tempting. So how can we consistently fit an intermittent fasting program into a life filled with jobs, kids, family get-togethers, and unpredictable stress?

Starting off slow is a good way to get used to an intermittent fasting program and get a feel for how it will fit into your life. It's okay to modify a fasting plan before jumping right into it, either by shortening the fasting period or increasing the number of calories eaten. For instance, if you want to try the 5:2 method but aren't sure about eating only 500 calories on fasting days, you could start off by eating 1000 calories on fasting days and slowly decrease them as you get used to the plan. Or start off by fasting only one day a week and see how it goes. If you want to try the 16:8 method but find the length of the fasting time a bit daunting, start with the 14:10 method and gradually increase the fasting time until you reach 16 hours.

You can also try a more flexible approach to your fasting program. With traditional fasting, your fasting schedule is exactly the same for each day or week. But if a rigid schedule doesn't work for you, it can easily be switched up depending on your needs. Say you're following the 16:8 method but have a hard time getting through the workday without food. During the week, your eating window could be from 10 a.m. to 6 p.m., helping to stave off hunger pangs at the office. But on weekends, when you may sleep in a bit longer and stay out a bit later, the window could be adjusted according to your weekend plans. And don't forget about dirty fasting – the few extra calories allowed in a dirty fast could be all you need to make it to your eating window. You can choose to dirty fast on days when you know you'll need a little extra calorie boost, but clean fast on other days. Being flexible with your fasting program can help it fit in with your lifestyle even if your schedule changes frequently.

Planning out a schedule for eating and fasting can also be helpful, especially if you know you have a busy week ahead. Figure out which times will work best for fasting and eating, and jot them down in a daily planner or spreadsheet. And speaking of planning, planning meals and snacks for the week can make intermittent fasting even easier. Many fasters enjoy prepping their weekly meals ahead of time, so they always have a healthy meal or snack on hand when it's time to eat. This way, when it's getting close to the end of your fast, you'll already know the answer to the question, "what should I eat?". Having a ready-to-eat meal on hand prevents the temptation of eating whatever is fastest, easiest, or cheapest, such as a vending machine candy bar or a burger and fries from a fast-food restaurant.

Running on Empty?

On its own, intermittent fasting can be a helpful tool to lose weight or stabilize blood sugar. But adding in some exercise to your weekly schedule is even more beneficial, no matter what your goals are. However, many fasters wonder how they should incorporate exercise into their fasting program. Should you exercise during a fast? Or wait until an eating window?

Before you decide when to exercise, there are some pros and cons to consider. Some experts believe that exercising during a fast can boost the benefits of both the exercise and the fast. As you fast, your body's carbohydrate stores, known as glycogen, are depleted. When you exercise, glycogen is one of the first things the body uses for fuel. But if glycogen has been depleted during a fasting period, the body must then turn to burning fat for energy. If you're trying to lose weight, this can provide some welcome motivation to stay consistent with your eating and exercise program.

But exercising during a fast may also cause your body to break down muscle in order to use protein for fuel. Since maintaining muscle is vital for keeping metabolism humming along smoothly, any muscle loss can hinder progress. One way to prevent this is by timing your exercise so that it occurs right before the end of your fast. As soon as you finish exercising, you can replenish your muscles by eating some healthy carbohydrates and protein.

Although exercising during a fast can be effective for some people, others find that they have less energy while fasting, making exercise more difficult. If trying to exercise on an empty stomach becomes a struggle, the healthy benefits of working up a sweat can be lost. In that case, it's better to save exercise for after a meal, when energy is high and your focus is sharp.

Of course, the most important thing to remember is that exercise should be a regular part of your life, whether you're fasting or not. When you exercise should not impact whether you exercise. In the same way, while there are pros and cons to exercising while fasting, whether or not you choose to wait for an eating window largely comes down to personal preference. In the end, the best time to exercise may simply be the time that fits into your schedule. Fasting or not, when you find a way to consistently fit exercise into your life, stick with it and make it a habit!

Getting Started

It can be a bit intimidating to embark on a new fasting program. After all, it means that you will be consciously and intentionally opting out of eating for a certain amount of time. In all likelihood, intermittent fasting will be a much different method of eating than you are used to. It may feel unnatural at first, and maybe even uncomfortable. And what about hunger pangs?

It's true that most of us will feel hungry now and then during fasting periods, but it's also important to remember that the feeling is fleeting, and nothing bad will happen if we feel hungry for a few minutes. Most hunger pangs last about 20 minutes, after which the feeling passes.

But perhaps even more challenging than true hunger is appetite, which is simply our desire to eat. Appetite can be fueled by emotions, like boredom and anxiety, or by our senses, such as smelling or seeing a delicious plate of food. It is also triggered by a hormone called ghrelin, which rises merely in anticipation of a meal. So if you eat at the same times every day, ghrelin levels are conditioned to rise at those times. This results in a "learned appetite" that tends to pop up at regular mealtimes, whether we are truly hungry or not. Powering through this "learned appetite" can be one of the most difficult parts of a new fasting program. The good news is, once your body readjusts to your new way of eating, the hunger and crankiness you might feel at first tends to dissipate. This can take between two and four weeks; but in the meantime, there are some strategies you can employ to make the transition between your usual way of eating and intermittent fasting easier.

To start a new intermittent fasting program on the right foot, begin preparation the night before with some good quality sleep. A good night's sleep sets the stage for the rest of your day, and this is especially important when embarking on a fasting program. Studies have shown that a lack of sleep causes an increase in the production of ghrelin, leading to feelings of hunger. Not to mention, we're less likely to exercise if we're feeling fatigued. Try to stick to a regular sleep schedule, and look for ways to wind down and relax at bedtime: keep your bedroom cool, avoid too much screen time, read a good book, or have a cup of calming herbal tea.

Since you may now be fasting at times when you're used to having a meal, try to distract yourself with other activities. Tackle a work project, meet up with friends for a (calorie-free) coffee, take a walk in nature, plan your next vacation—anything that will keep boredom from creeping in. Boredom, much like fatigue, can easily lead to food cravings and a desire to eat called "psychological hunger." This can happen even if we're not truly hungry; but fasting presents the challenge of true physical hunger as well, making it even more important to stay busy and prevent boredom.

And don't discount the importance of staying hydrated while fasting. Drinking plenty of water, along with other non-caloric beverages like tea or coffee, is a simple but effective way to stay on track with an intermittent fasting program. Water, even with its zero-calorie nutrition profile, can trick the brain into thinking the stomach is full, staving off hunger until it's time to break the fast. It's a good idea to always keep a water bottle on hand, especially if you often forget to sip water or if you're out running errands.

Finally, when you do break your fast, eat slowly and mindfully, eating every few hours during the eating window. It can be tempting, of course, to dive right into a huge meal after a long fasting period, but remember that eating too much will negate the positive effects of the fast. You want to gradually ingest your day's worth of calories during the eating window, without going overboard and indulging too much. Some experts also recommend adding a few tablespoons of a healthy fat, such as olive oil or avocado, to your last meal of the day.

This helps to keep blood sugar steady as you move into the next fasting period.

Carbs, Fats, and Fiber

The most important part of intermittent fasting may not be the fasting itself, but rather the food you eat when you're not fasting. While there are really no "rules" when it comes to what you can and can't eat during an intermittent fasting program, you'll see more progress and reap more benefits if you eat a healthy diet. It wouldn't make much sense to expend all that effort fasting only to end up indulging in chips, ice cream, and cookies after every fast! Remember, you're not fasting so you can eat junk food; you're fasting for specific goals like weight loss or lowering blood sugar, and these can not be achieved with a poor, high-calorie diet, even combined with fasting.

In fact, eating a healthy diet is even more important during intermittent fasting, because restricting your eating means you have less time to make sure you're ingesting all the vitamins and key nutrients you need in a day. During eating windows, your focus should be on nutrient-dense foods like vegetables, fruits, whole grains, and lean protein.

There are some specific types of foods that are especially valuable when fasting, which can help you achieve your goals. First and foremost is the ubiquitous beverage that has already been mentioned (but is definitely worth repeating): water. Ask just

about any nutritionist or dietitian for their most recommended food to eat during an intermittent fast and they'll no doubt say "water." Of course, it's not technically a "food," but it's a vital component of your intermittent fasting toolbox.

Next, aim to eat some good-quality, complex carbohydrates. Some of us have been taught to believe that carbohydrates are the "enemy" when it comes to losing weight or eating healthy, but this simply isn't true. While you don't want to go overboard on high-calorie foods like French fries or mac and cheese, eating minimally processed carbohydrates like whole-grain bread, potatoes, black beans, and chickpeas gives you quick energy and is an easily digestible fuel source for your body.

Another food group with a "bad" reputation is fats; but when eaten in moderation, many fats are actually very beneficial and can even help with weight loss. Foods like avocados, nuts, olive oil, and ghee help to keep you full longer with a minimal amount of calories. Studies show that fats help to trigger feelings of satiety, even if you haven't filled up on food. Eating just half an avocado with a meal helps to keep you full for hours longer than if you ate the same meal without the avocado. Thanks to these satiating properties, fats can be especially helpful to eat with your last meal of the day, as you head into a long fasting period.

Fiber-rich foods are important to include during your mealtimes, as well. These include vegetables like broccoli, Brussels sprouts, and greens; fruits like raspberries, pears, and apples; grains like barley, quinoa, and oatmeal; and legumes like peas, lentils, and black beans. Many of us fall short of eating enough fiber in our diets, and we're missing out on its many health benefits. In addition to keeping digestion running smoothly, fiber helps to lower cholesterol and blood sugar. And, since high-fiber foods are more filling than low-fiber foods, you can eat less but still feel full. That makes high-fiber foods ideal for an intermittent fasting program.

Lean meats, fish, eggs, and dairy can round out your intermittent fasting diet, but of course you can adapt your food choices to reflect your own eating style. The beauty of an intermittent fasting program is that any style of eating—vegetarian, vegan, low-carb, paleo, keto—can fit into your new lifestyle. You simply eat the diet of your choice during your eating window. Intermittent fasting's flexibility makes it a perfect program for just about anyone!

Make Your Calories Count

Just as there are foods you should aim to eat during your eating window, there are also some foods it is best to avoid when you break your fast. Try to stay away from fast food, sugar, refined starches, trans fats, and processed foods like luncheon meats or boxed cereals. And whereas water is an obvious given when it comes to beverages, it's best to avoid sweet drinks like fruit juices and sodas. These sorts of foods and drinks don't pack much nutritional punch, but they do pack calories. And the last thing you want during an intermittent fasting program is empty calories.

What's more, foods that are high in sugar or contain highly processed carbohydrates not only don't have the satiating properties of nutrients like protein and healthy fats, but they also digest quickly and increase levels of the hunger hormone ghrelin, resulting in cravings for more sugary foods. You may have noticed this effect after eating candy or a bag of potato chips. Chances are, you only felt satisfied by the snack for a short amount of time. An hour later, you may have been searching the fridge and pantry again, looking for more sugary or starchy foods.

Eating the right kinds of foods is essential to reaching your goals with an intermittent fasting program. While an occasional piece of cake or a slice of pizza, eaten in moderation, won't sabotage your overall progress, continued bad eating habits will definitely hinder your results. It may be true that all calories have the same amount of energy—4.184 joules, to be precise—but as we've seen, not all calories are created equal. When you're participating in any kind of fasting program, you need the calories you eat to count toward giving your body the nutrition it needs.

As you begin your journey with intermittent fasting, remember to ease into the program slowly to get used to the fasting process. Plan your days so you know when you'll be fasting and when you'll be eating. Prepare some healthy meals and snacks ahead of time so you're ready to tackle your new lifestyle without distractions and temptations. And, most importantly, stay consistent with whichever intermittent fasting method you choose. Before you know it, you'll begin to see and feel changes, giving you the motivation to continue on your journey.

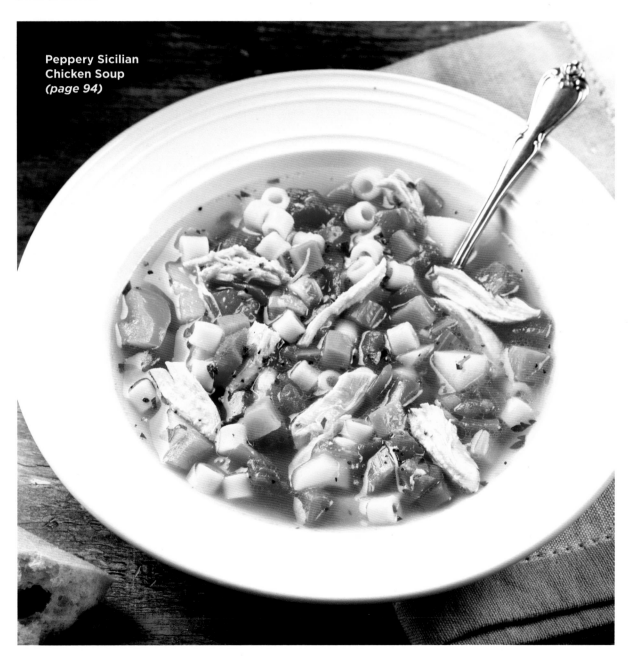

Peppery Sicilian Chicken Soup *(page 94)*

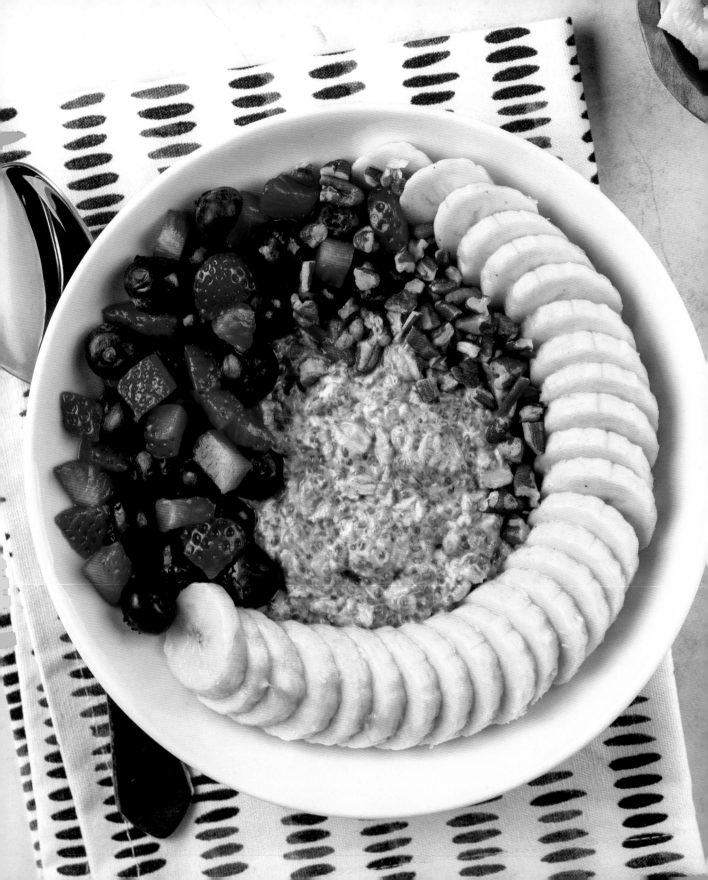

BREAKFAST

Overnight Chia Oat Pudding

1 cup old-fashioned oats

¼ cup chia seeds

3 tablespoons palm sugar or packed brown sugar, divided

½ teaspoon ground cinnamon

½ teaspoon salt

1¾ cups oatmilk

1 cup fresh strawberries, stemmed and diced

1 cup fresh blueberries

4 tablespoons chopped pecans or sliced almonds

4 bananas, sliced (optional)

1 Combine oats, chia seeds, 2 tablespoons sugar, cinnamon and salt in medium bowl or food storage container. Add oatmilk; stir until well blended. Cover and refrigerate overnight.

2 Combine strawberries and remaining 1 tablespoon sugar in small bowl or food storage container. Cover and refrigerate overnight.

3 Stir oat mixture. Stir blueberries into strawberries. For each serving, scoop ½ cup oat mixture into bowl. Top with berry mixture and pecans. Serve with bananas, if desired.

MAKES 4 SERVINGS

½ CUP PUDDING, ¼ OF BERRIES AND 1 TABLESPOON NUTS PER SERVING:

calories 340

total fat 16g

saturated fat 4g

sodium 400mg

carbs 45g

fiber 11g

sugar 22g

protein 10g

Avocado Toast

½ cup thawed frozen peas

2 teaspoons lemon juice

1 teaspoon minced fresh tarragon

¼ teaspoon plus ⅛ teaspoon salt, divided

⅛ teaspoon black pepper

1 teaspoon olive oil

1 tablespoon pepitas (raw pumpkin seeds)

4 slices hearty whole grain bread, toasted

1 avocado

1 Combine peas, lemon juice, tarragon, ¼ teaspoon salt and pepper in small food processor; pulse until blended but still chunky. Or combine all ingredients in small bowl and mash with fork to desired consistency.

2 Heat oil in small saucepan over medium heat. Add pepitas; cook and stir 1 to 2 minutes or until toasted. Transfer to small bowl; stir in remaining ⅛ teaspoon salt.

3 Spread about 1 tablespoon pea mixture over each slice of toast. If making one serving, place the remaining pea mixture in a jar or container and store in the refrigerator for a day or two.

4 Cut avocado in half lengthwise around pit. If making one serving, wrap the half with the pit in plastic wrap and store in the refrigerator for 1 day. Cut the avocado into slices in the shell; use a spoon to scoop the slices out of the shell. Arrange avocado slices on top of pea mixture; top with toasted pepitas.

MAKES 2 SERVINGS

2 TOASTS PER SERVING:

calories 380

total fat 22g

saturated fat 4g

sodium 680mg

carbs 37g

fiber 9g

sugar 6g

protein 13g

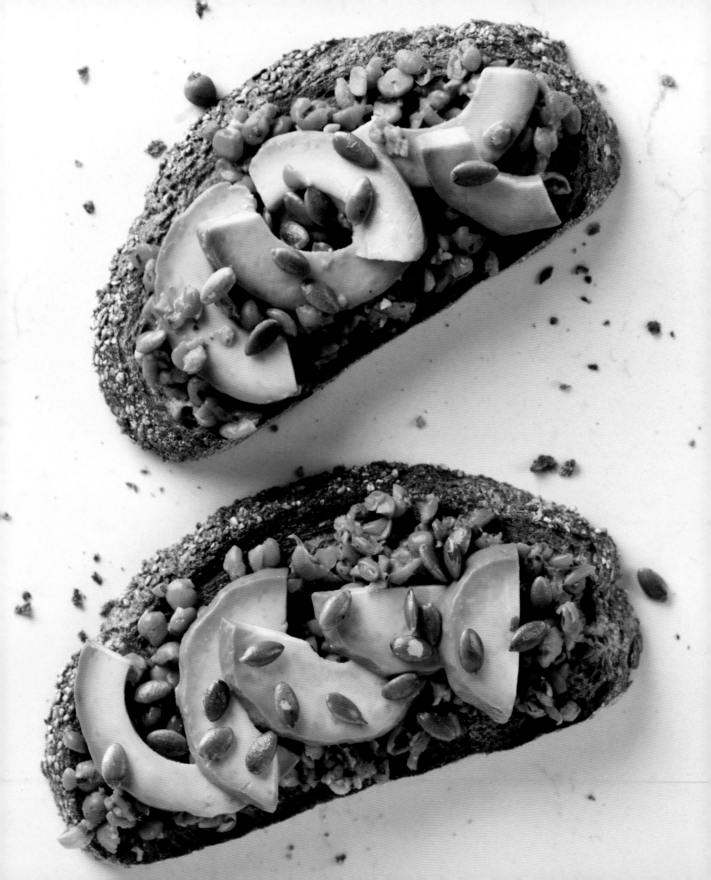

Vegetable Quinoa Frittata

1 tablespoon olive oil

1 cup chopped onion

1 cup small broccoli florets

¾ cup finely chopped red bell pepper

2 cloves garlic, minced

1¼ teaspoons coarse salt

Black pepper

1½ cups cooked quinoa (see Note)

¼ cup sun-dried tomatoes (not packed in oil), chopped

8 eggs, lightly beaten

¼ cup grated Parmesan cheese

1 Preheat oven to 400°F.

2 Heat oil in large ovenproof nonstick skillet over medium-high heat. Add onion and broccoli; cook and stir 4 minutes, Add bell pepper; cook and stir 2 minutes. Add garlic, salt and black pepper; cook 30 seconds, stirring constantly. Stir in quinoa and sun-dried tomatoes.

3 Pour eggs over quinoa mixture in skillet; stir gently to mix. Cook 3 to 5 minutes or until eggs are set around edge, lifting edge to allow uncooked portion to flow underneath. Sprinkle with cheese.

4 Bake about 7 minutes or until eggs are set. Let stand 5 minutes; cut into six wedges.

NOTE: For cooked quinoa, rinse ¾ cup uncooked quinoa in fine-mesh strainer under cold water. Bring 1½ cups water, quinoa and 1 teaspoon salt, if desired, to a boil in medium saucepan. Reduce heat to low; cover and simmer 10 to 15 minutes or until quinoa is tender and water is absorbed.

MAKES 6 SERVINGS

1 WEDGE PER SERVING:

calories **220**

total fat **11g**

saturated fat **4g**

sodium **580mg**

carbs **16g**

fiber **3g**

sugar **4g**

protein **14g**

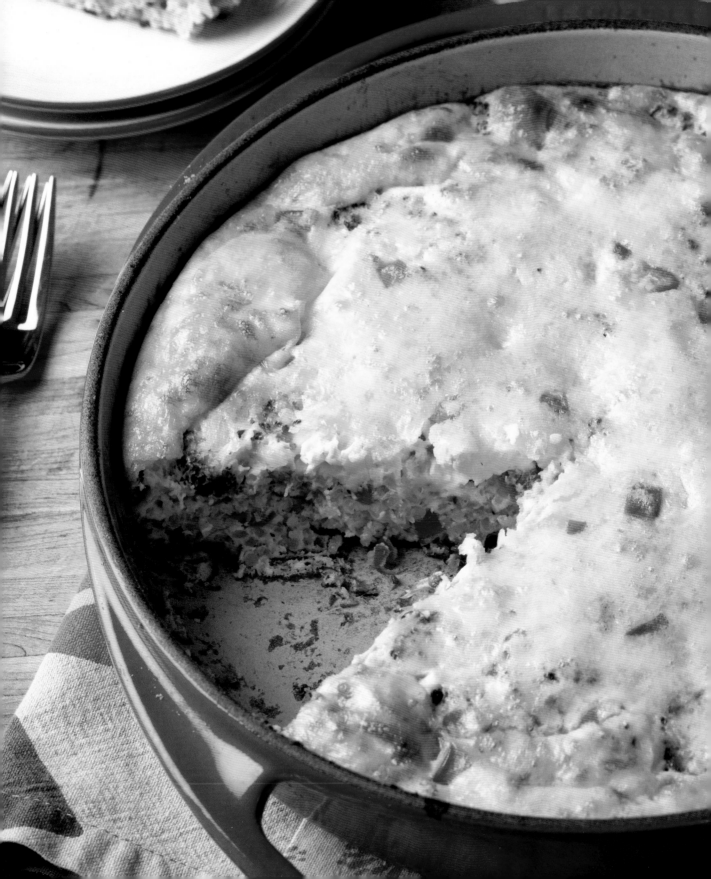

Oatmeal with Apples and Cottage Cheese

⅔ **cup water**

¼ **teaspoon salt**

½ **cup old-fashioned oats**

½ **cup diced apple**

2 **tablespoons packed brown sugar, granulated sugar or raw sugar**

1 **teaspoon vanilla**

¾ **teaspoon ground cinnamon**

½ **cup cottage cheese**

¼ **cup half-and-half**

2 **tablespoons chopped pecans or almonds**

1 Bring water and salt to a boil in small saucepan over high heat. Stir in oats, apple, sugar, vanilla and cinnamon. Reduce heat to medium-low; cook and stir 3 to 5 minutes or until oats are tender and creamy.

2 Stir in cottage cheese and half-and-half; spoon into serving bowls. Top with nuts.

MAKES 2 SERVINGS

½ OF TOTAL RECIPE PER SERVING:

calories 270

total fat 8g

saturated fat 2g

sodium 470mg

carbs 36g

fiber 4g

sugar 20g

protein 12g

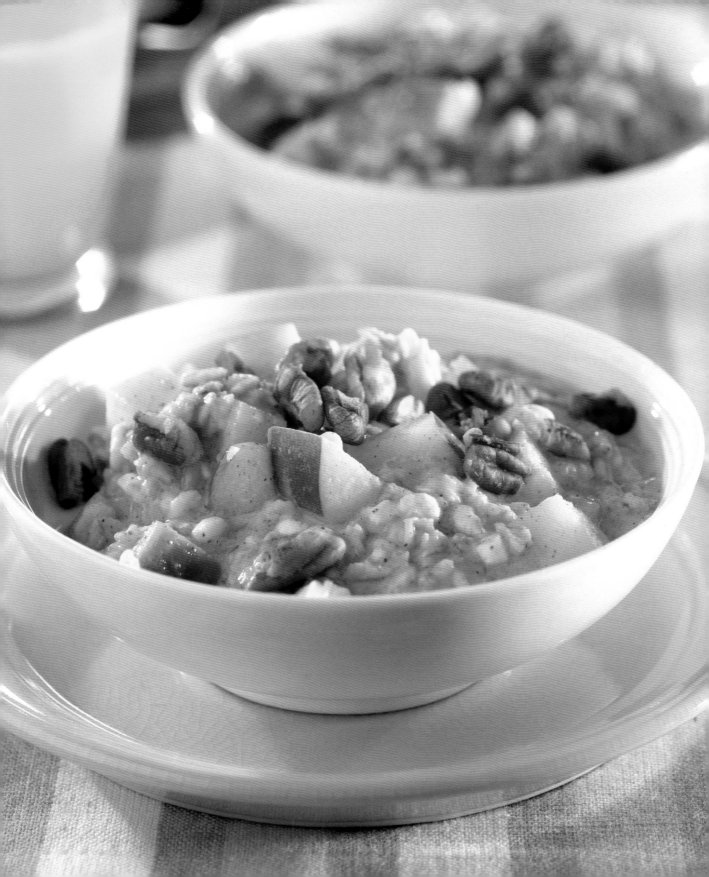

Frittata Rustica

4 ounces cremini
  mushrooms, stems
  trimmed, cut into
  thirds

1 tablespoon olive oil,
  divided

½ teaspoon plus
  ⅛ teaspoon salt,
  divided

½ cup chopped onion

1 cup packed
  chopped stemmed
  lacinato kale

½ cup halved grape
  tomatoes

4 eggs

½ teaspoon Italian
  seasoning

  Black pepper

⅓ cup shredded
  mozzarella cheese

1 tablespoon
  shredded
  Parmesan cheese

  Chopped fresh
  parsley (optional)

1 Preheat oven to 400°F. Spread mushrooms on small baking sheet; drizzle with 1 teaspoon oil and sprinkle with ⅛ teaspoon salt. Roast 15 to 20 minutes or until well browned and tender.

2 Heat remaining 2 teaspoons oil in small (6- to 8-inch) ovenproof nonstick skillet over medium heat. Add onion; cook and stir 5 minutes or until softened. Add kale and ¼ teaspoon salt; cook and stir 10 minutes or until kale is tender. Add tomatoes; cook and stir 3 minutes or until tomatoes are soft. Stir in mushrooms.

3 Preheat broiler. Whisk eggs, remaining ¼ teaspoon salt, Italian seasoning and pepper in small bowl until well blended.

4 Pour egg mixture over vegetables in skillet; stir gently to mix. Cook 3 minutes or until eggs are set around edge, lifting edge to allow uncooked portion to flow underneath. Sprinkle with mozzarella and Parmesan.

5 Broil 3 minutes or until eggs are set and cheese is browned. Cut into wedges; garnish with parsley.

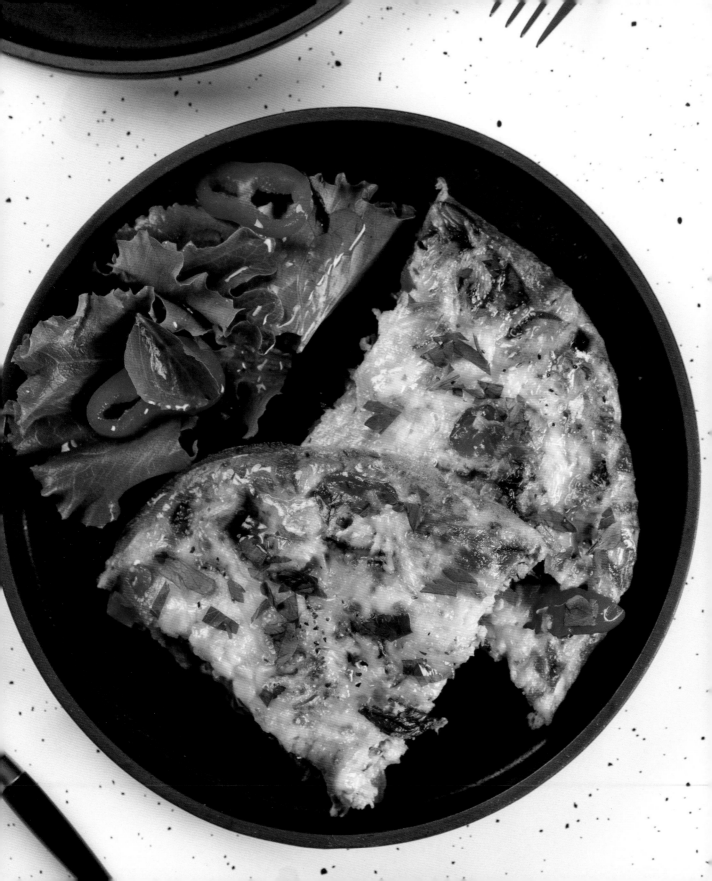

Banana Split Breakfast Bowl

2½ **tablespoons sliced almonds**

2½ **tablespoons chopped walnuts**

3 **cups vanilla nonfat Greek yogurt**

1⅓ **cups sliced fresh strawberries (about 12 medium)**

2 **bananas, cut in half and sliced lengthwise**

½ **cup drained pineapple tidbits**

1 Spread almonds and walnuts in single layer in small heavy skillet. Cook and stir over medium heat 2 minutes or until lightly browned. Immediately remove from skillet; cool completely.

2 Spoon yogurt into four bowls. Top with strawberries, banana slices and pineapple. Sprinkle with toasted nuts.

MAKES 4 SERVINGS

1 BOWL PER SERVING:

calories 240

total fat 5g

saturated fat 0g

sodium 50mg

carbs 37g

fiber 4g

sugar 25g

protein 14g

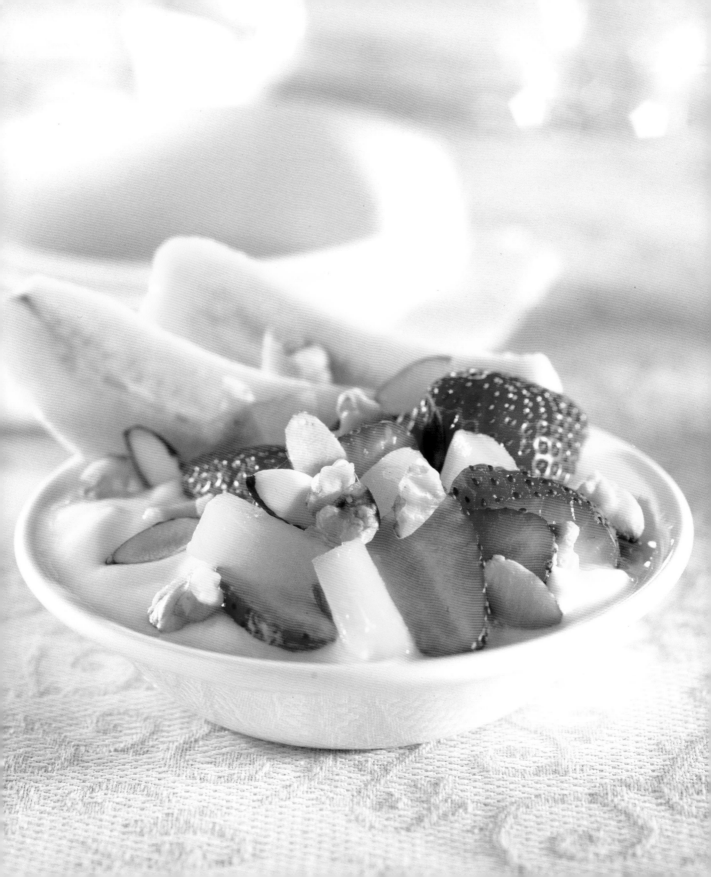

Crisp Oats Trail Mix

- **1 cup old-fashioned oats**
- **½ cup pepitas (raw pumpkin seeds)**
- **2 tablespoons maple syrup**
- **1 teaspoon canola oil**
- **½ teaspoon ground cinnamon**
- **¼ teaspoon salt**
- **½ cup dried sweetened cranberries**
- **½ cup raisins**

1 Preheat oven to 325°F. Line baking sheet with foil.

2 Combine oats, pepitas, maple syrup, oil, cinnamon and salt in large bowl; mix well. Spread on prepared baking sheet.

3 Bake 20 minutes or until oats are lightly browned, stirring once. Cool completely on baking sheet. Stir in cranberries and raisins. Store in airtight container.

TIP: Serve this trail mix with plain yogurt and fresh berries or pack it in small containers to munch on the go.

MAKES 2½ CUPS (ABOUT 10 SERVINGS)

¼ CUP PER SERVING:

calories 123

total fat 5g

saturated fat 1g

sodium 60mg

carbs 20g

fiber 2g

sugar 11g

protein 3g

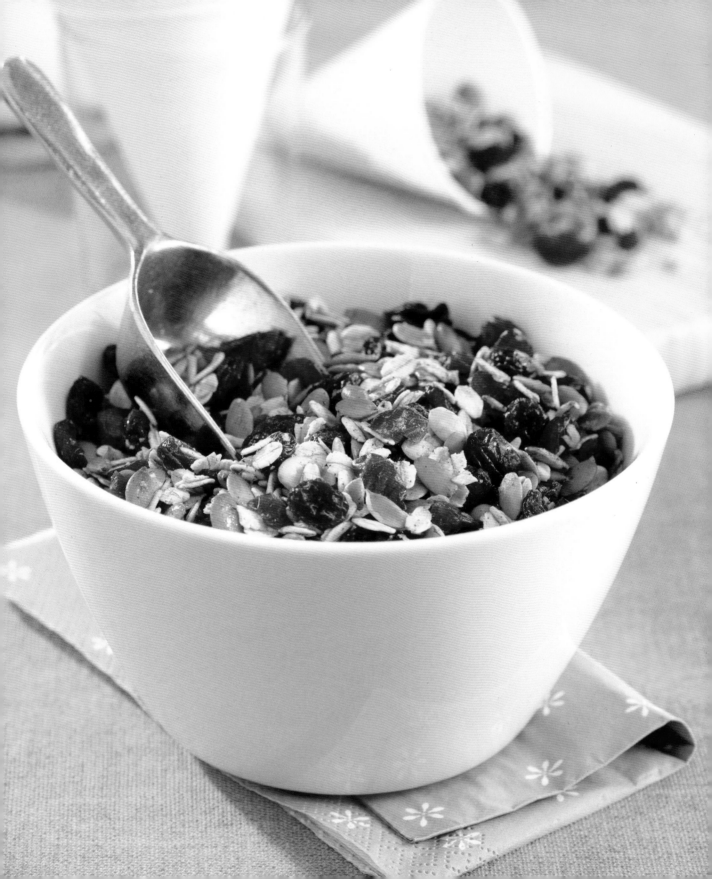

Mini Spinach Frittatas

1 tablespoon olive oil

½ cup chopped onion

8 eggs

¼ cup plain yogurt

1 package
  (10 ounces) frozen
  chopped spinach,
  thawed and
  squeezed dry

½ cup (2 ounces)
  shredded white
  Cheddar cheese

¼ cup grated
  Parmesan cheese

¾ teaspoon salt

⅛ teaspoon black
  pepper

⅛ teaspoon ground
  red pepper

  Dash ground
  nutmeg

1 Preheat oven to 350°F. Spray 12 standard (2½-inch) muffin cups with nonstick cooking spray.

2 Heat oil in small nonstick skillet over medium heat. Add onion; cook and stir about 5 minutes or until softened. Set aside to cool slightly.

3 Whisk eggs and yogurt in large bowl. Stir in spinach, Cheddar, Parmesan, salt, black pepper, red pepper, nutmeg and onion until blended. Divide mixture evenly among prepared muffin cups.

4 Bake 20 to 25 minutes or until eggs are puffed and firm and no longer shiny. Cool in pan 2 minutes. Loosen bottom and sides with small spatula or knife; remove to wire rack. Serve warm, cold or at room temperature.

MAKES 12 MINI FRITTATAS

3 FRITTATAS PER SERVING:

calories 290

total fat 20g

saturated fat 8g

sodium 850mg

carbs 6g

fiber 2g

sugar 2g

protein 21g

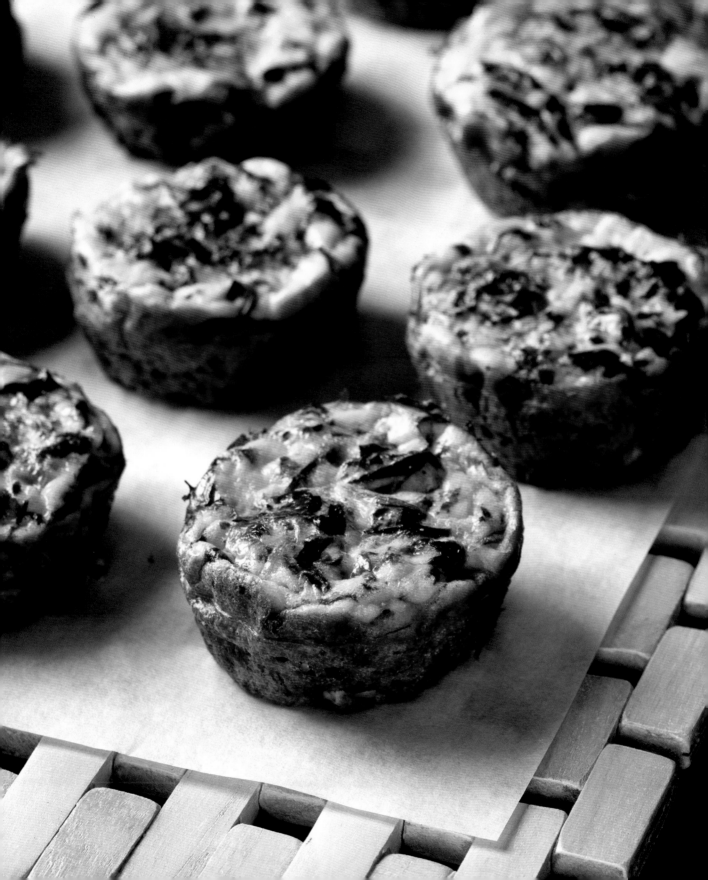

Fruity Whole-Grain Cereal

2 cups water

½ teaspoon salt

¼ cup uncooked quick-cooking pearl barley

¼ cup uncooked instant brown rice

½ cup soymilk or almond milk

⅓ cup golden raisins

¼ cup finely chopped dried dates

¼ cup chopped dried plums

¼ cup old-fashioned oats

¼ cup oat bran

2 tablespoons packed brown sugar

½ teaspoon ground cinnamon

1 Bring water and salt to a boil in medium saucepan. Add barley and rice. Reduce heat to low; cover and simmer 8 minutes.

2 Stir in soymilk, raisins, dates, plums, oats, oat bran, brown sugar and cinnamon. Cover and simmer 10 minutes or until mixture is creamy and grains are al dente, stirring once. Serve hot.

TIP: To reheat leftover cereal, place one serving in microwavable bowl. Microwave 30 seconds; stir. Add water or milk to reach desired consistency. Microwave just until hot.

MAKES 4 SERVINGS

¼ OF TOTAL RECIPE PER SERVING:

calories 210

total fat 2g

saturated fat 0g

sodium 310mg

carbs 50g

fiber 5g

sugar 24g

protein 5g

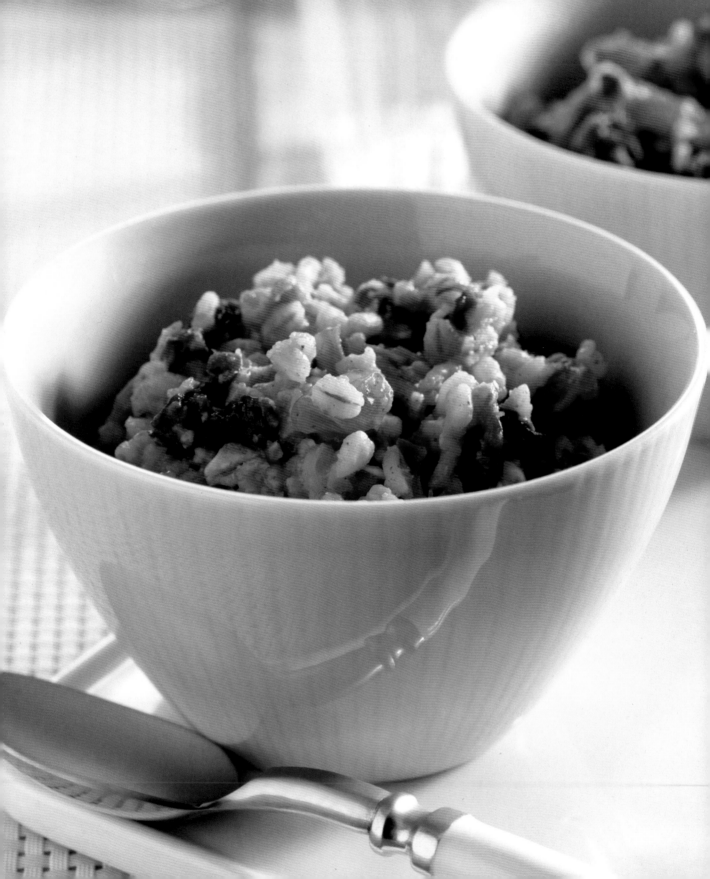

Smoked Salmon Omelet

3 **eggs**

2 **tablespoons milk**

1 **tablespoon grated Parmesan cheese**

Pinch white or black pepper

1 **teaspoon butter**

2 **tablespoons finely chopped red onion, divided**

1 **ounce smoked salmon, cut into 1- to 2-inch pieces**

2 **tablespoons sour cream**

1 **tablespoon water**

1 **tablespoon capers, rinsed and drained**

Finely chopped fresh parsley (optional)

1 Whisk eggs, milk, cheese and pepper in small bowl until well blended.

2 Heat butter in small (6-inch) nonstick skillet over medium-high heat. Pour egg mixture into skillet; stir briefly. Let eggs begin to set at edges, then lift edges and tilt skillet, allowing uncooked portion of egg mixture to flow underneath. Cook 1 minute or until omelet begins to set. Sprinkle 1 tablespoon onion over half of omelet; top with smoked salmon. Fold other half of omelet over filling; cook 1 minute. Slide omelet onto serving plate.

3 Whisk sour cream and water in small bowl until blended. Drizzle over omelet; top with remaining 1 tablespoon onion, capers and parsley, if desired.

MAKES 1 SERVING

1 OMELET PER SERVING:

calories **400**

total fat **28g**

saturated fat **13g**

sodium **1070mg**

carbs **6g**

fiber **1g**

sugar **4g**

protein **29g**

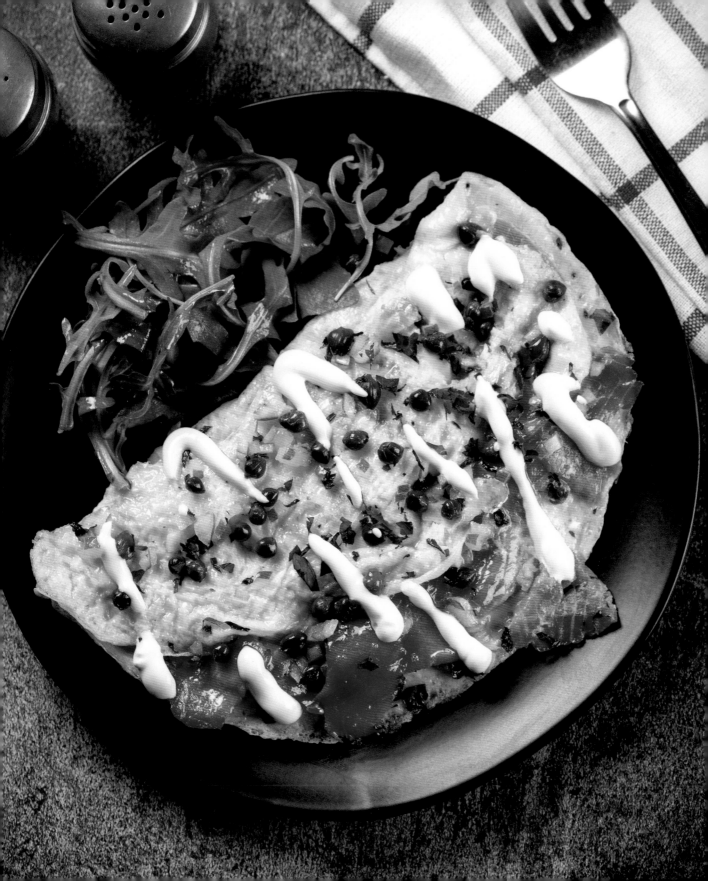

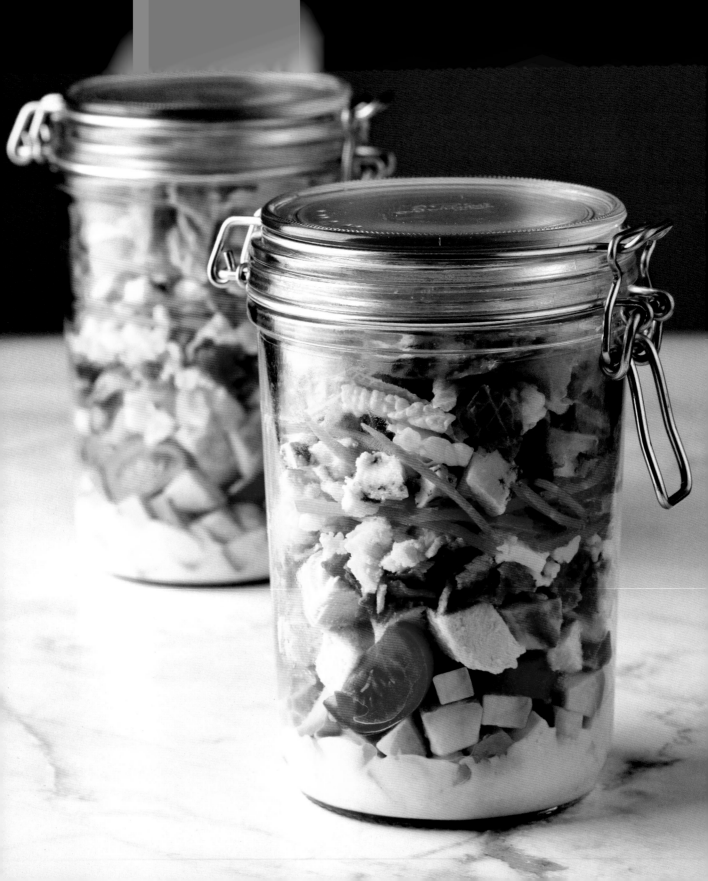

LUNCHES

Cobb Salad to Go

½ **cup blue cheese salad dressing**

1 **ripe avocado, diced**

1 **tomato, chopped**

6 **ounces cooked chicken breast, cut into 1-inch pieces**

4 **slices bacon, crisp-cooked and crumbled**

2 **hard-cooked eggs, mashed with fork**

1 **large carrot, shredded**

½ **cup crumbled blue cheese**

1 **package (10 ounces) torn mixed salad greens**

1 Place 2 tablespoons salad dressing in bottom of four (1-quart) jars. Layer remaining ingredients on top, ending with salad greens. Seal jars.

2 Refrigerate until ready to serve. To serve, shake salad until well blended or pour into a bowl and stir to mix.

MAKES 4 SERVINGS

1 SALAD PER SERVING:

calories 440

total fat 33g

saturated fat 8g

sodium 790mg

carbs 12g

fiber 6g

sugar 4g

protein 25g

Curried Chicken Wraps

⅓ cup mayonnaise

2 tablespoons mango chutney

½ teaspoon curry powder

4 (6-inch) corn tortillas

1½ cups shredded coleslaw mix

1½ cups shredded or chopped cooked chicken

2 tablespoons chopped lightly salted peanuts

1 tablespoon chopped fresh cilantro

1 Combine mayonnaise, chutney and curry powder in small bowl; mix well. Spread evenly onto one side of each tortilla.

2 Top evenly with coleslaw mix, chicken, peanuts and cilantro. Roll up to enclose filling.

MAKES 4 SERVINGS

1 WRAP PER SERVING:

calories 380

total fat 24g

saturated fat 4g

sodium 420mg

carbs 20g

fiber 3g

sugar 2g

protein 21g

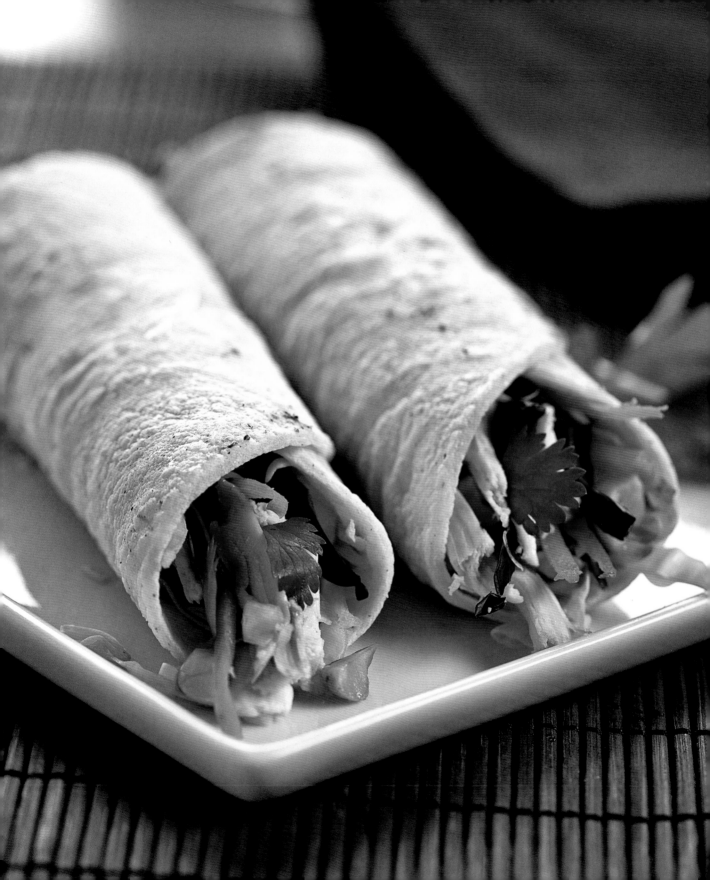

Mediterranean Tuna Sandwiches

MAKES 4 SERVINGS

1 SANDWICH
(2 HALVES)
PER SERVING:

calories 340

total fat 11g

saturated
fat 2g

sodium
460mg

carbs 32g

fiber 3g

sugar 6g

protein 28g

- 1 can (12 ounces) solid white tuna packed in water, drained
- ¼ cup finely chopped red onion
- ¼ cup fat-free or reduced-fat mayonnaise
- 3 tablespoons chopped black olives, drained
- 1 tablespoon plus 1 teaspoon lemon juice
- 1 tablespoon chopped fresh mint (optional)
- 1 tablespoon olive oil
- ¼ teaspoon black pepper
- ⅛ teaspoon garlic powder (optional)
- 8 slices whole wheat bread
- 8 romaine lettuce leaves
- 8 thin slices tomato

1 Combine tuna, onion, mayonnaise, olives, lemon juice, mint, if desired, oil, pepper and garlic powder, if desired, in large bowl until blended.

2 Top each of four slices bread with lettuce leaves and tomato slices. Top with tuna mixture and remaining bread slices. Cut sandwiches in half to serve.

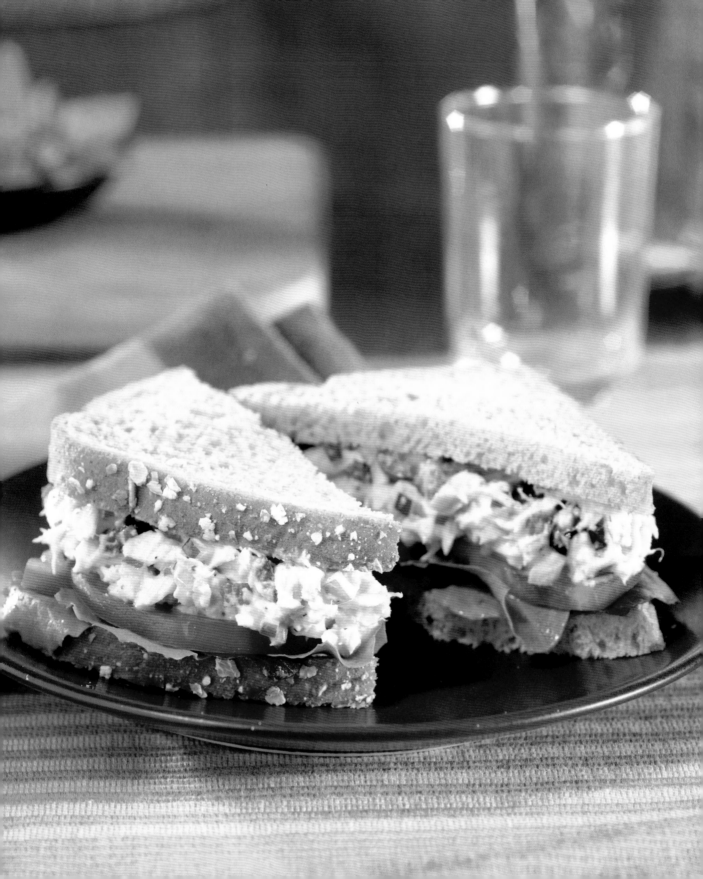

Grilled Baja Burritos

6 tablespoons vegetable oil, divided

3 tablespoons lime juice, divided

2 teaspoons chili powder

1½ teaspoons lemon-pepper

1 pound tilapia fillets

3 cups coleslaw mix

½ cup chopped fresh cilantro

¼ teaspoon salt

¼ teaspoon black pepper

Guacamole and pico de gallo (optional)

4 (6-inch) flour tortillas

Lime wedges (optional)

1 Prepare grill for direct cooking or preheat broiler. Combine 2 tablespoons oil, 1 tablespoon lime juice, chili powder and lemon-pepper in large resealable food storage bag. Add fish; seal bag and turn to coat. Let stand at room temperature 10 minutes.

2 Brush grid with 2 tablespoons oil. Remove fish from marinade; discard marinade. Grill fish, covered, over medium-high heat 6 to 8 minutes or until center is opaque, carefully turning once. (To broil, place 4 inches away from heat source. Broil 3 to 5 minutes per side or until center is opaque.)

3 Combine coleslaw mix, remaining 2 tablespoons oil, 2 tablespoons lime juice, cilantro, salt and pepper in medium bowl; mix well.

4 Layer fish, coleslaw mixture, guacamole and pico de gallo, if desired, on tortillas. Fold up about 1 inch of bottom and top of tortilla; roll up from one side to enclose filling. Serve with additional pico de gallo and lime wedges, if desired.

TIP: Any firm white fish, such as snapper or halibut, would make a great substitute for the tilapia.

MAKES 4 SERVINGS

1 BURRITO PER SERVING:

calories 430
total fat 26g
saturated fat 5g
sodium 680mg
carbs 25g
fiber 3g
sugar 1g
protein 27g

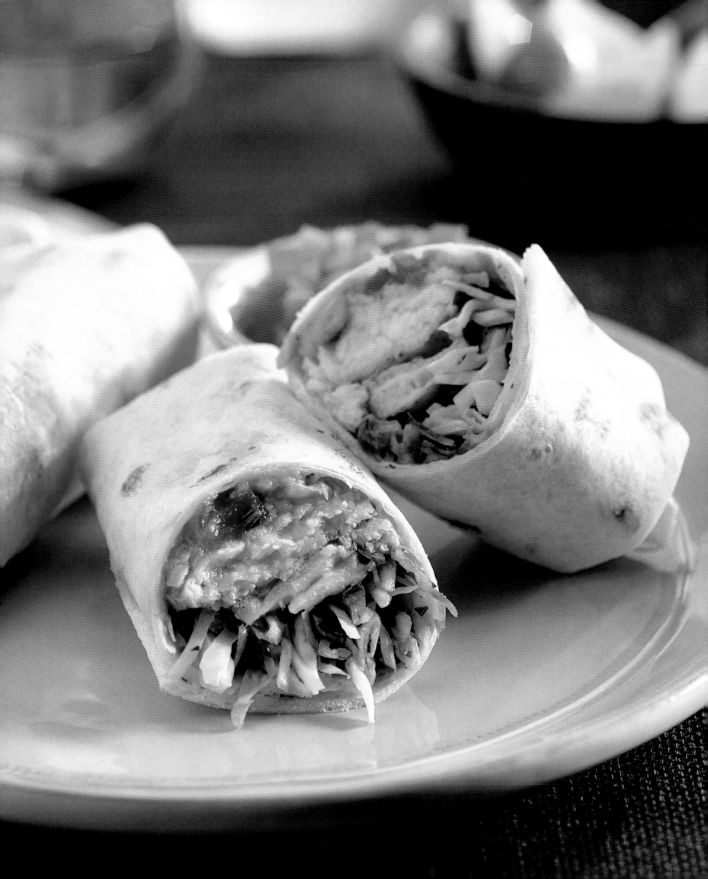

Greek Chicken Burgers with Cucumber Yogurt Sauce

½ **cup plus 2 tablespoons plain nonfat Greek yogurt**

½ **medium cucumber, peeled, seeded and finely chopped**

Juice of ½ lemon

3 **cloves garlic, minced, divided**

2 **teaspoons finely chopped fresh mint** *or* ½ **teaspoon dried mint**

⅛ **teaspoon salt**

⅛ **teaspoon ground white pepper**

1 **pound ground chicken**

¾ **cup (3 ounces) crumbled reduced-fat feta cheese**

4 **large kalamata olives, pitted and minced**

1 **egg**

½ **teaspoon dried oregano**

¼ **teaspoon black pepper**

Mixed greens (optional)

1 Combine yogurt, cucumber, lemon juice, 2 cloves garlic, chopped mint, salt and white pepper in medium bowl; mix well. Cover and refrigerate until ready to serve.

2 Combine chicken, cheese, olives, egg, oregano, black pepper and remaining 1 clove garlic in large bowl; mix well. Shape mixture into four patties.

3 Spray grill pan with nonstick cooking spray; heat over medium-high heat. Grill patties 5 to 7 minutes per side or until cooked through (165°F).

4 Serve burgers with sauce and mixed greens, if desired.

MAKES 4 SERVINGS

1 BURGER AND ¼ OF SAUCE PER SERVING:

calories 270

total fat 12g

saturated fat 4g

sodium 430mg

carbs 4g

fiber 1g

sugar 3g

protein 31g

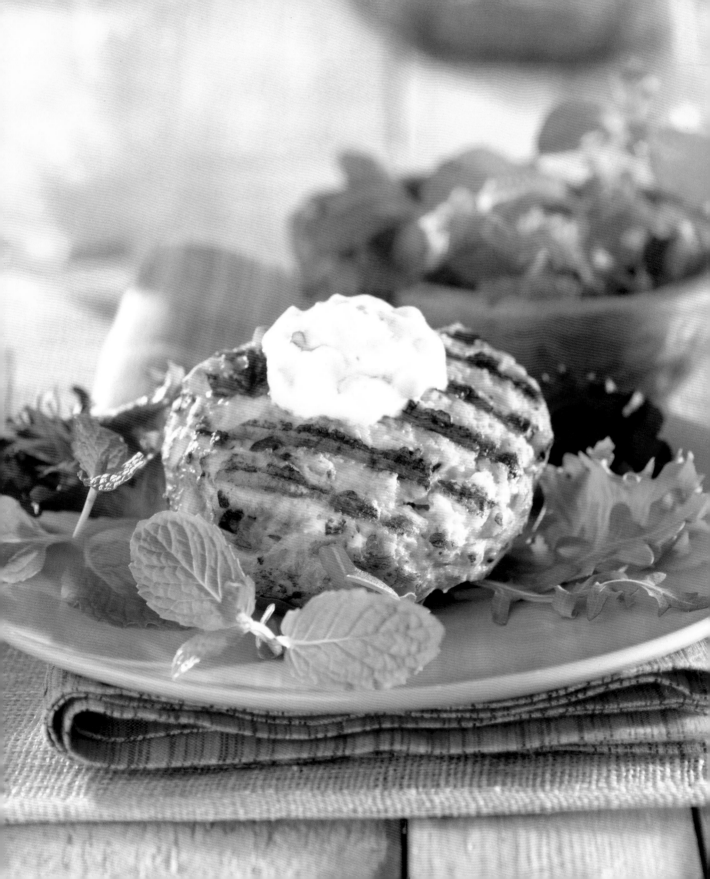

Stuffed Turkey Pitas with Cranberry Mustard and Blue Cheese

½ **cup whole berry cranberry sauce**

2 **to 3 tablespoons coarse grain mustard**

8 **ounces chopped cooked turkey breast (about 1 cup)**

4 **pita breads, cut in half crosswise**

4 **cups packed spring greens (about 3½ ounces)**

½ **cup thinly sliced red onion**

½ **cup crumbled blue cheese**

1 Whisk cranberry sauce and mustard in small bowl until well blended. Add turkey; stir to coat evenly.

2 Fill each pita half with equal amounts greens, turkey mixture, onion and cheese.

TIP: This is a great use for leftover Thanksgiving turkey. If you don't have turkey, use packaged cooked chicken or a rotisserie chicken.

MAKES 4 SERVINGS

2 STUFFED PITA HALVES PER SERVING:

calories 370

total fat 8g

saturated fat 4g

sodium 730mg

carbs 49g

fiber 1g

sugar 12g

protein 19g

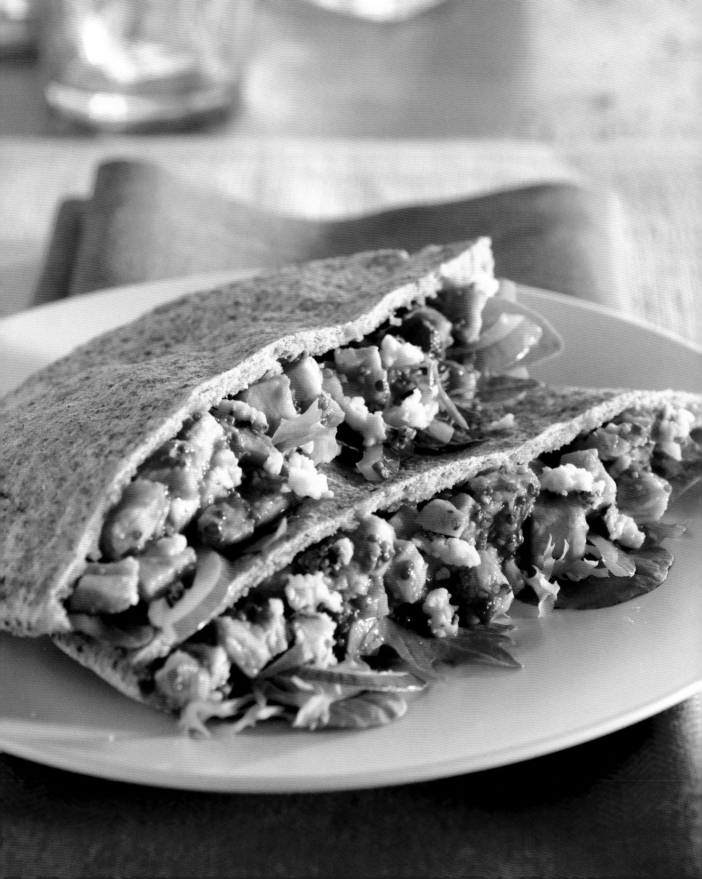

Chicken and Quinoa Bowl

MAKES 4 SERVINGS

1 BOWL PER SERVING:

calories 550

total fat 31g

saturated fat 5g

sodium 800mg

carbs 38g

fiber 8g

sugar 5g

protein 34g

1 cup uncooked quinoa

2 cups water

1¼ teaspoons salt, divided

1 large ripe avocado

1 teaspoon lime juice

2 tablespoons finely chopped red onion

1 tablespoon chopped fresh cilantro

2 teaspoons minced jalapeño pepper

4 boneless skinless chicken breasts (4 to 6 ounces each)

¾ teaspoon black pepper, divided

5 tablespoons olive oil, divided

3 tablespoons lemon juice

1 pint cherry tomatoes, halved

1 seedless cucumber, thinly sliced

Optional toppings: arugula, sliced radishes, sliced red cabbage, lemon wedges and/or black sesame seeds

1 Rinse quinoa in fine-mesh strainer under cold water. Combine 2 cups water, quinoa and ½ teaspoon salt in medium saucepan. Bring to a boil over high heat. Reduce heat to low; cover and simmer 10 to 15 minutes or until quinoa is tender and water is absorbed. Transfer to large bowl; cool to room temperature.

2 Cut avocado in half lengthwise around pit; remove pit. Scoop avocado into medium bowl; sprinkle with lime juice and toss to coat. Mash to desired consistency with fork or potato masher. Add onion, cilantro, jalapeño and ¼ teaspoon salt; stir gently until well blended.

3 Meanwhile, season chicken with remaining ½ teaspoon salt and ½ teaspoon black pepper. Heat 1 tablespoon oil in large skillet over medium-high heat. Cook chicken about 10 minutes or until lightly browned and no longer pink in center (165°F), turning once. Transfer to cutting board; slice chicken.

4 Whisk remaining 4 tablespoons oil, lemon juice and remaining ¼ teaspoon black pepper in small bowl until well blended. Stir into quinoa.

5 Divide quinoa mixture among four bowls or food storage containers. Top with tomatoes, cucumber, chicken and avocado mixture. Serve with desired toppings.

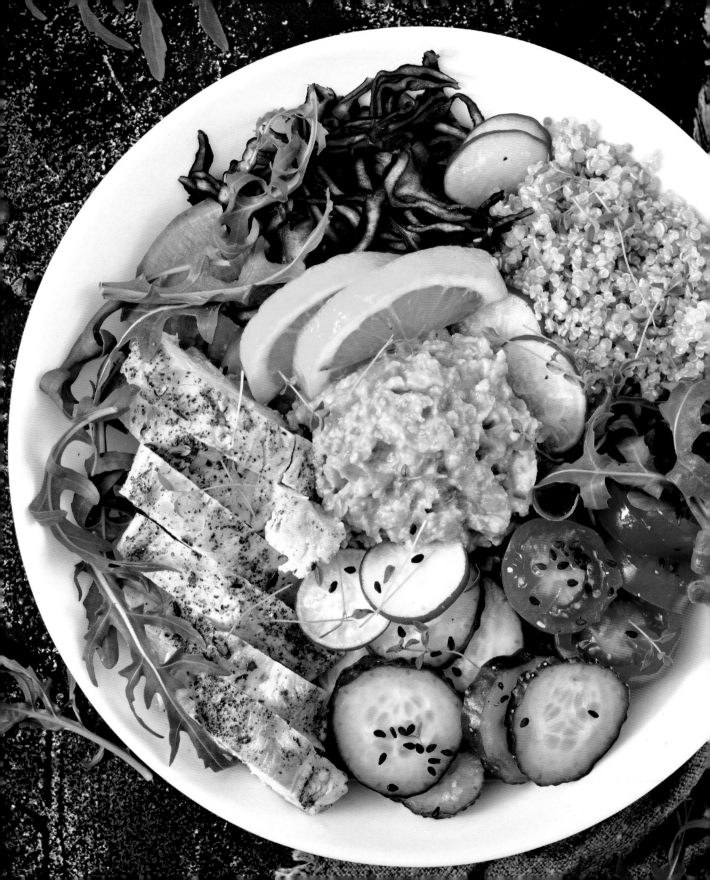

Mediterranean Sandwiches

1¼ **pounds chicken tenders, cut crosswise in half**

1 **large tomato, diced**

½ **small cucumber, halved lengthwise, seeded and sliced**

½ **cup sweet onion slices**

2 **tablespoons cider vinegar**

1 **tablespoon olive or canola oil**

1 **tablespoon minced fresh oregano *or* ½ teaspoon dried oregano**

2 **teaspoons minced fresh mint *or* ¼ teaspoon dried mint**

¼ **teaspoon salt**

6 **(6-inch) whole wheat pita breads, cut in half crosswise**

1 Spray large nonstick skillet with nonstick cooking spray; heat over medium heat. Add chicken; cook and stir 7 to 10 minutes or until browned and cooked through. Let stand 5 to 10 minutes to cool slightly.

2 Combine chicken, tomato, cucumber and onion in medium bowl. Add vinegar, oil, oregano, mint and salt; toss to coat. Refrigerate until ready to serve.

3 Divide chicken mixture evenly among pita halves.

MAKES 6 SERVINGS

2 FILLED PITA HALVES PER SERVING:

calories 450

total fat 18g

saturated fat 4g

sodium 950mg

carbs 54g

fiber 1g

sugar 5g

protein 21g

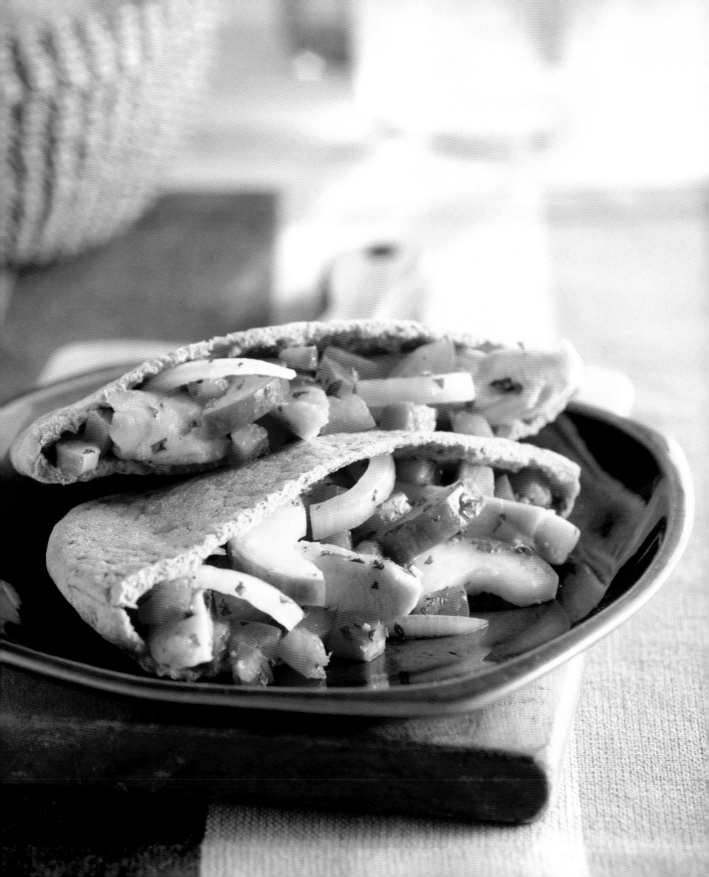

Spinach Veggie Wraps

PICO DE GALLO

- **1 cup finely chopped tomatoes (about 2 small)**
- **½ teaspoon salt**
- **¼ cup chopped white onion**
- **2 tablespoons minced jalapeño pepper**
- **2 tablespoons chopped fresh cilantro**
- **1 teaspoon lime juice**

GUACAMOLE

- **2 large ripe avocados**
- **¼ cup finely chopped red onion**
- **2 tablespoons chopped fresh cilantro**
- **2 teaspoons lime juice**
- **½ teaspoon salt**

WRAPS

- **4 (10-inch) whole wheat tortillas**
- **2 cups fresh baby spinach leaves**
- **1 cup sliced mushrooms**
- **1 cup shredded Asiago cheese**
- **Salsa**

1 For pico de gallo, combine tomatoes and ½ teaspoon salt in fine-mesh strainer; set over bowl to drain 15 minutes. Combine drained tomatoes, white onion, jalapeño, 2 tablespoons cilantro and 1 teaspoon lime juice in medium bowl; mix well.

2 For guacamole, combine avocados, red onion, 2 tablespoons cilantro, 2 teaspoons lime juice and ½ teaspoon salt in medium bowl; mash with fork to desired consistency.

3 For wraps, spread ¼ cup guacamole on each tortilla. Layer each with ½ cup spinach, ¼ cup mushrooms, ¼ cup cheese and ¼ cup pico de gallo. Roll up; serve with salsa.

TIP: To make these wraps super easy, purchase premade pico de gallo and guacamole from the grocery store.

MAKES 4 SERVINGS

1 WRAP PER SERVING:

calories 410
total fat 27g
saturated fat 8g
sodium 920mg
carbs 34g
fiber 9g
sugar 7g
protein 14g

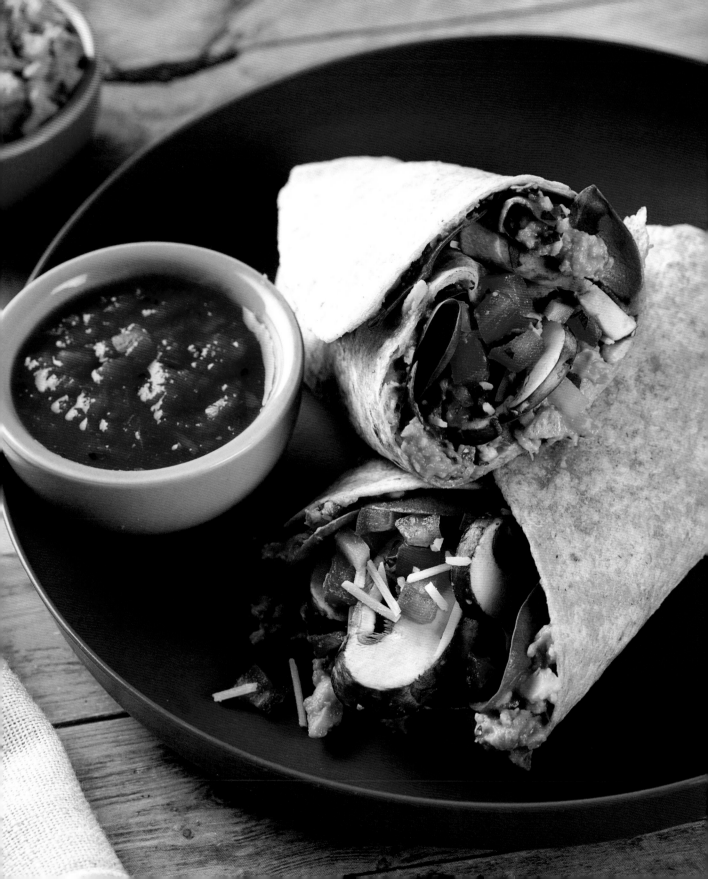

Roasted Cauliflower Salad in Pitas

- 1 **large head cauliflower (2½ pounds), cut into 1-inch florets**
- 2 **tablespoons olive oil**
- ¾ **teaspoon salt, divided**
- ¼ **teaspoon black pepper**
- ½ **cup mayonnaise**
- ¼ **cup plain Greek yogurt**
- 1 **teaspoon cider vinegar**
- 1 **teaspoon Dijon mustard**
- 1 **cup red grapes, halved**
- 2 **tablespoons minced fresh chives**
- ½ **cup chopped walnuts, toasted**
- 3 **pita breads, halved**
  Lettuce or microgreens

1 Preheat oven to 425°F. Place cauliflower on large baking sheet. Drizzle with oil and sprinkle with ½ teaspoon salt and pepper; toss to coat. Roast 45 minutes or until cauliflower is well browned and very tender. Cool completely.

2 Whisk mayonnaise, yogurt, vinegar, mustard and remaining ¼ teaspoon salt in large bowl. Stir in grapes, chives and cauliflower. Fold in walnuts. Line pita halves with lettuce; stuff with salad.

MAKES 6 SERVINGS

1 FILLED PITA HALF PER SERVING:

calories 360
total fat 25g
saturated fat 4g
sodium 630mg
carbs 33g
fiber 5g
sugar 10g
protein 9g

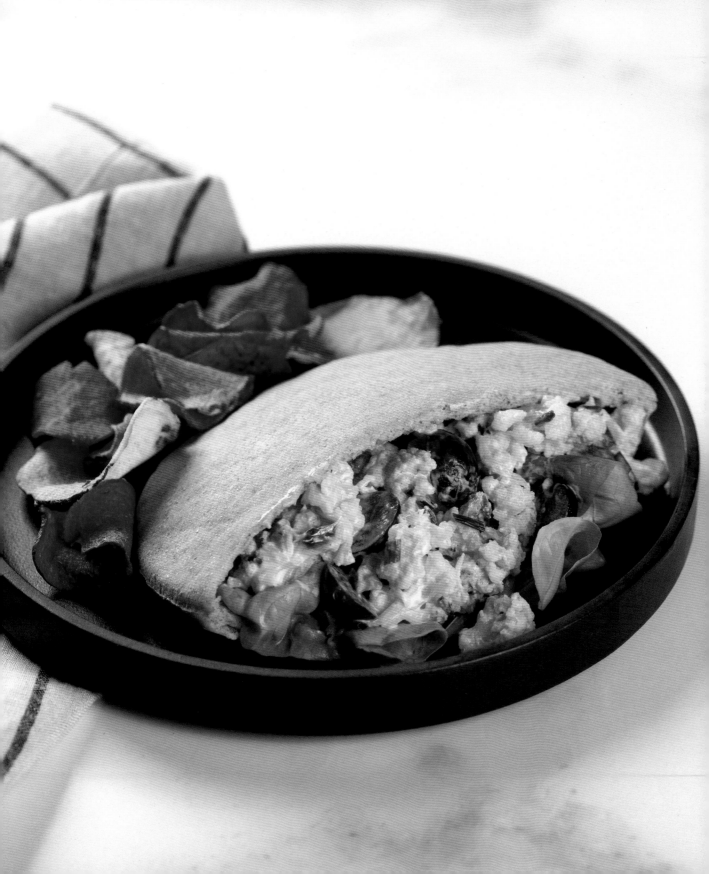

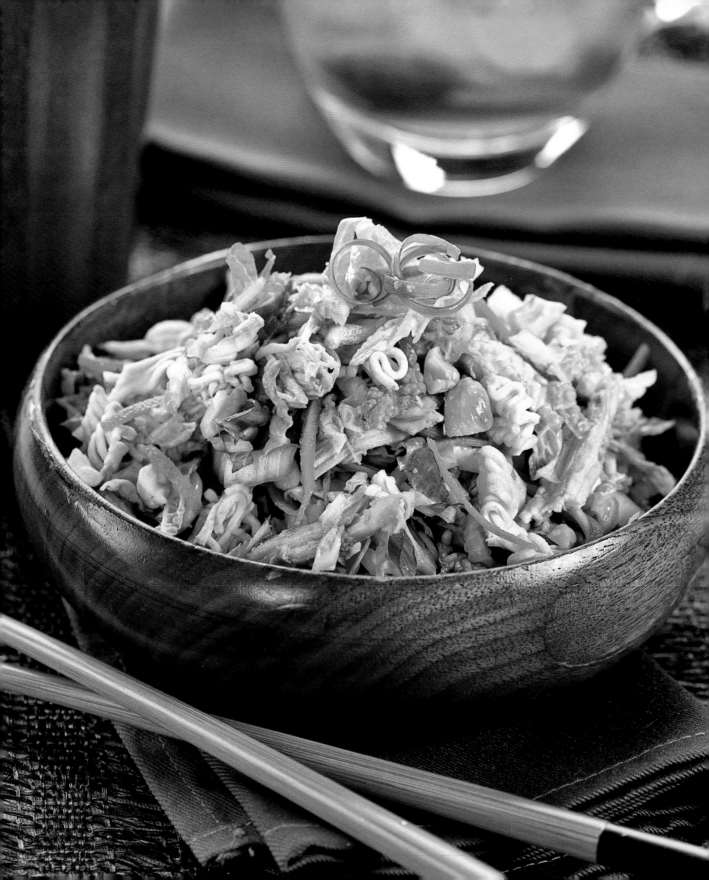

SALADS

Chinese Chicken Salad

- 3 tablespoons peanut or vegetable oil
- 3 tablespoons rice vinegar
- 2 tablespoons soy sauce
- 1 tablespoon honey
- 1 teaspoon minced fresh ginger
- 1 teaspoon toasted sesame oil
- 1 clove garlic, minced
- ¼ teaspoon red pepper flakes (optional)
- 4 cups shredded cooked chicken or turkey
- 4 cups packed shredded napa cabbage or romaine lettuce
- 1 cup shredded carrots
- ½ cup thinly sliced green onions
- 1 package (3 ounces) ramen noodles, crumbled* *or* 1 can (5 ounces) chow mein noodles
- ¼ cup chopped cashew nuts or peanuts (optional)

Use any flavor; discard seasoning packet.

1 For dressing, combine peanut oil, vinegar, soy sauce, honey, ginger, sesame oil, garlic and red pepper flakes, if desired, in small jar with tight-fitting lid; shake well.

2 Place chicken in large bowl. Pour dressing over chicken; toss to coat.**

3 Add cabbage, carrots, green onions and crumbled noodles to bowl; toss well to coat. Sprinkle with cashews, if desired.

**Salad may be made ahead to this point; cover and refrigerate chicken mixture until ready to serve.

MAKES 6 SERVINGS

¹/₆ OF TOTAL RECIPE PER SERVING:

calories 320

total fat 14g

saturated fat 3g

sodium 1240mg

carbs 17g

fiber 1g

sugar 7g

protein 30g

Warm Salmon Salad

DRESSING

⅓ **cup vegetable oil**

¼ **cup red wine vinegar**

2 **tablespoons finely chopped fresh chives**

2 **tablespoons finely chopped fresh parsley**

⅛ **teaspoon salt**

⅛ **teaspoon white pepper**

SALAD

2 **cups water**

¼ **cup chopped onion**

2 **tablespoons red wine vinegar**

¼ **teaspoon black pepper**

Salt

1¼ **pounds small red potatoes**

1 **pound salmon steaks**

6 **cups torn washed mixed salad greens**

2 **medium tomatoes, cut into wedges**

16 **pitted kalamata olives, sliced**

1 For dressing, combine oil, ¼ cup vinegar, chives, parsley, salt and white pepper in jar with tight-fitting lid; shake well to combine. Refrigerate until ready to use.

2 Combine water, onion, 2 tablespoons vinegar, black pepper and a large pinch of salt in large saucepan; bring to a boil over medium-high heat. Add potatoes. Reduce heat to medium-low; cover and cook 10 minutes or until fork-tender. Transfer potatoes to cutting board with slotted spoon; cool slightly. Reserve water in saucepan.

3 Cut potatoes into thick slices; place in medium bowl. Toss with ⅓ cup dressing.

4 Rinse salmon and pat dry with paper towels. To poach fish, place in reserved water and simmer gently 4 to 5 minutes or until fish is opaque and begins to flake easily when tested with fork. *Do not boil.* Carefully remove fish to cutting board with slotted spatula. Let stand 5 minutes; remove skin and bones. Cut fish into 1-inch pieces.

5 Divide salad greens among four plates; top with fish, potatoes, tomatoes and olives. Drizzle with remaining dressing.

MAKES 4 SERVINGS

¼ OF TOTAL RECIPE PER SERVING:

calories 570

total fat 38g

saturated fat 6g

sodium 450mg

carbs 30g

fiber 5g

sugar 5g

protein 28g

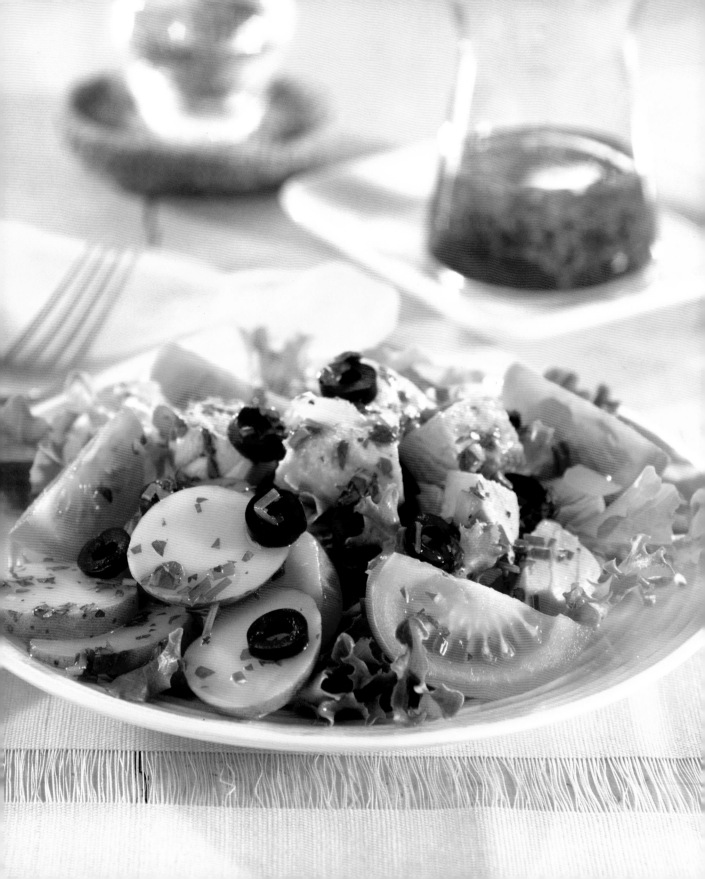

Strawberry Chicken Salad

DRESSING

- **1 cup fresh strawberries, hulled**
- **½ cup vegetable oil**
- **6 tablespoons white wine vinegar**
- **3 tablespoons sugar**
- **3 tablespoons honey**
- **2 tablespoons balsamic vinegar**
- **2 teaspoons Dijon mustard**
- **½ teaspoon dried oregano**
- **¼ teaspoon salt**

SALAD

- **4 cups chopped romaine lettuce**
- **4 cups coarsely chopped fresh spinach**
- **1 cup sliced fresh strawberries**
- **½ cup walnuts, toasted***
- **½ cup crumbled feta cheese**
- **2 cups warm cooked chicken slices (about half of a rotisserie chicken)** *or* **12 ounces grilled chicken breast strips**

  See Note on page 64.

1 For dressing, combine whole strawberries, oil, white wine vinegar, sugar, honey, balsamic vinegar, mustard, oregano and salt in blender or food processor; blend 30 seconds or until smooth.

2 For each salad, combine 1 cup lettuce and 1 cup spinach on serving plate; top with ¼ cup sliced strawberries, 2 tablespoons walnuts and 2 tablespoons cheese. Top with chicken; drizzle with dressing.

TIP: To make this salad extra special, substitute glazed walnuts for the plain walnuts. Glazed walnuts can be found in the produce section of the supermarket along with other salad toppings, or they may be found in the snack or baking aisles. Or, to make your own, see the Tip on page 74.

MAKES 6 SERVINGS

$\frac{1}{6}$ OF TOTAL RECIPE PER SERVING:

calories 440

total fat 30g

saturated fat 5g

sodium 560mg

carbs 24g

fiber 3g

sugar 20g

protein 22g

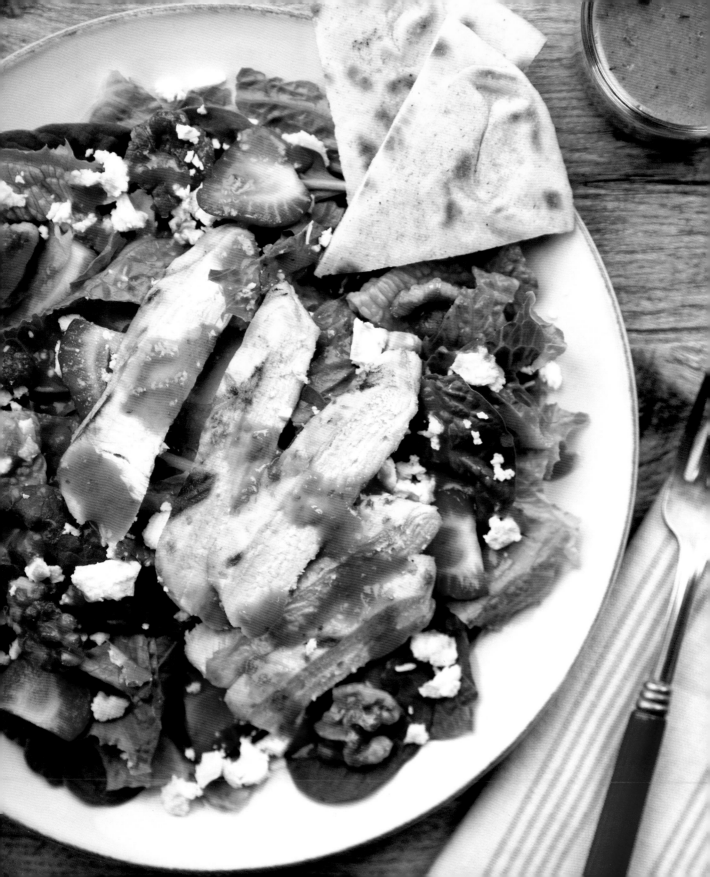

Taco Salad

1 **pound 90% lean ground beef or turkey**

1 **small onion, finely chopped**

1 **clove garlic, minced**

2 **teaspoons chili powder**

1 **teaspoon ground cumin**

½ **teaspoon salt**

Dash black pepper

1 **large head iceberg lettuce, cut into bite-size pieces (about 10 cups)**

2 **large tomatoes, chopped**

1 **medium avocado, sliced**

2 **cups salsa (optional)**

1 Brown ground beef in medium skillet over medium-high heat 6 to 8 minutes, stirring to break up meat. Drain fat. Add onion and garlic; cook and stir about 5 minutes or until onion is softened. Stir in chili powder, cumin and salt.

2 Divide lettuce, tomatoes and avocado among serving plates; top with ground beef mixture. Serve with salsa, if desired.

MAKES 4 SERVINGS

¼ OF TOTAL RECIPE PER SERVING:

calories 330
total fat 19g
saturated fat 6g
sodium 440mg
carbs 16g
fiber 7g
sugar 7g
protein 26g

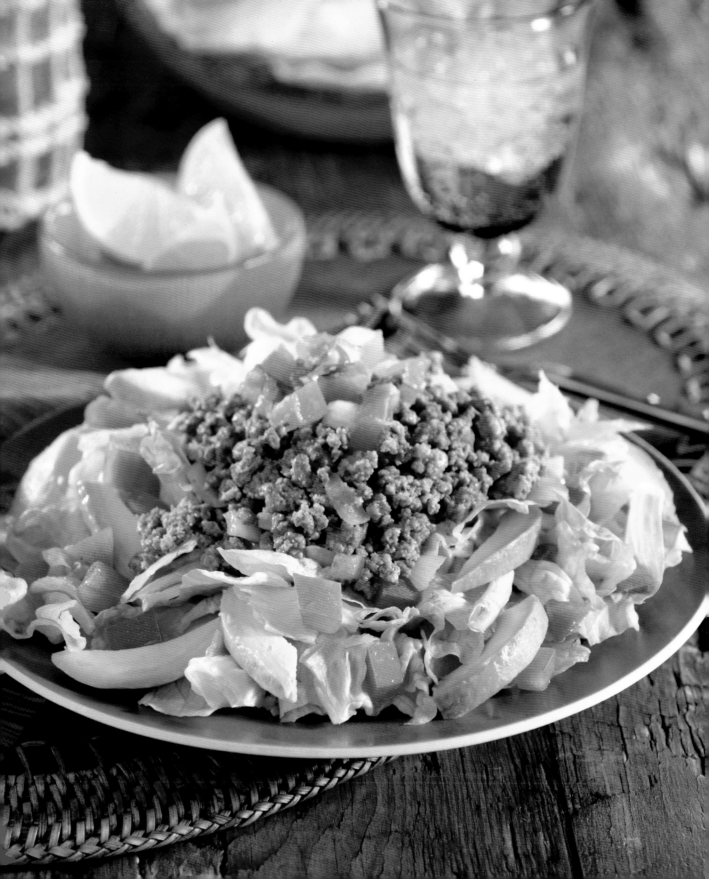

Amazing Apple Salad

DRESSING

- **5 tablespoons apple juice concentrate**
- **¼ cup white balsamic vinegar**
- **1 tablespoon lemon juice**
- **1 tablespoon sugar**
- **1 clove garlic, minced**
- **½ teaspoon salt**
- **½ teaspoon onion powder**
- **¼ teaspoon ground ginger**
- **¼ cup olive oil**

SALAD

- **12 cups mixed greens such as chopped romaine lettuce and spring greens**
- **12 ounces thinly sliced cooked chicken**
- **2 tomatoes, cut into wedges**
- **1 package (about 3 ounces) dried apple chips**
- **½ red onion, thinly sliced**
- **½ cup crumbled gorgonzola or blue cheese**
- **½ cup pecans, toasted (see Note)**

1 For dressing, whisk apple juice concentrate, vinegar, lemon juice, sugar, garlic, salt, onion powder and ginger in small bowl until blended. Slowly whisk in oil in thin, steady stream until well blended.

2 For salad, divide greens among four serving bowls. Top with chicken, tomatoes, apple chips, onion, cheese and pecans.

3 Drizzle about 2 tablespoons dressing over each salad.

NOTE: To toast pecans, cook in medium skillet over medium heat 3 to 4 minutes or until lightly browned and fragrant, stirring frequently.

MAKES 4 SERVINGS

¼ OF TOTAL RECIPE PER SERVING:

calories 630

total fat 36g

saturated fat 6g

sodium 920mg

carbs 46g

fiber 6g

sugar 34g

protein 34g

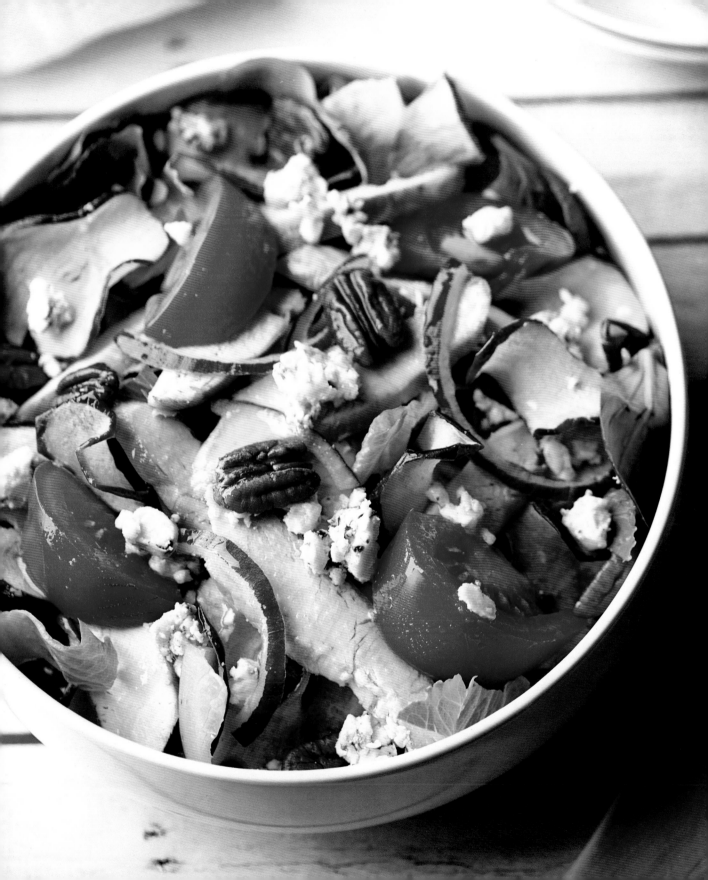

Chicken Satay Salad

¼ cup plus
  2 tablespoons
  Thai peanut sauce,
  divided

2 tablespoons lime
  juice

1 tablespoon
  unseasoned rice
  vinegar

3 teaspoons toasted
  sesame oil, divided

1 pound chicken
  tenders, cut in half
  lengthwise

4 cups chopped
  romaine lettuce

1 red bell pepper,
  thinly sliced

1 cup shredded carrots

1 cup sliced Persian* or
  seedless cucumbers

¼ cup chopped fresh
  cilantro

1 tablespoon peanuts,
  chopped

*Persian cucumbers
are similar to seedless
(English) cucumbers;
they have fewer seeds
and contain less
water than traditional
cucumbers, which gives
them a sweeter flavor
and crunchier texture.
These smaller cucumbers
can be found in packages
in the produce section of
the supermarket.*

1 Whisk ¼ cup peanut sauce, lime juice, vinegar and 1 teaspoon oil in large bowl until smooth and well blended.

2 Heat remaining 2 teaspoons oil in large nonstick skillet over medium-high heat. Add chicken; cook and stir 4 minutes or until chicken is no longer pink. Remove from heat. Add remaining 2 tablespoons peanut sauce; gently toss to coat evenly.

3 Add lettuce, bell pepper, carrots and cucumbers to dressing in large bowl; toss to coat.

4 Divide salad evenly among four plates. Top with chicken, cilantro and peanuts.

MAKES 4 SERVINGS

¼ OF TOTAL RECIPE PER SERVING:

calories 265
total fat 10g
saturated fat 1g
sodium 643mg
carbs 14g
fiber 3g
sugar 8g
protein 28g

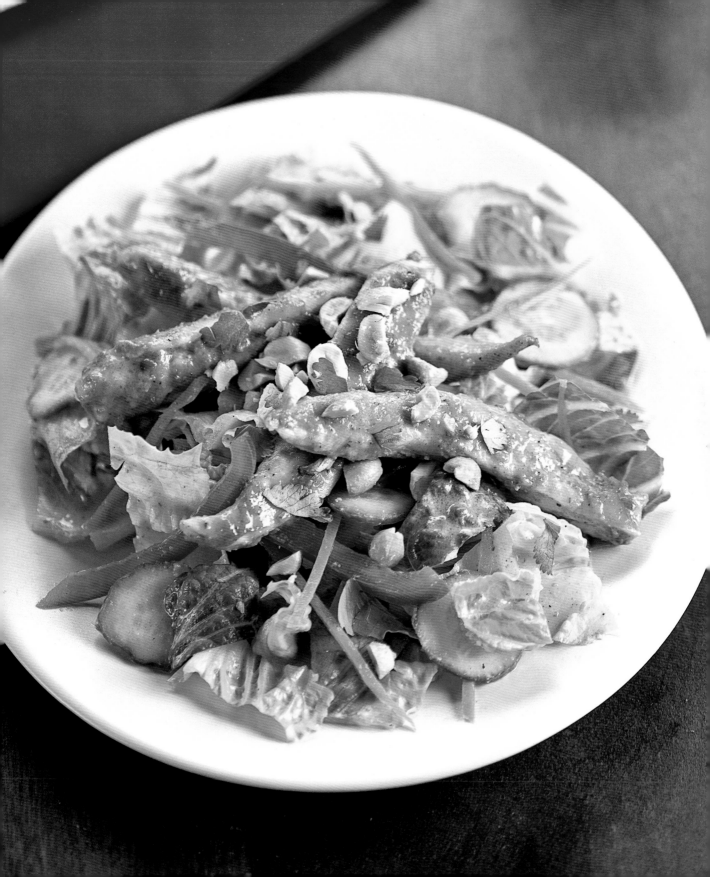

Sweet Italian Marinated Vegetable Salad

DRESSING

- **2 tablespoons white or rice wine vinegar**
- **1 tablespoon chopped fresh oregano *or* 1 teaspoon dried oregano**
- **2 teaspoons sugar**
- **⅛ teaspoon salt**
- **⅛ teaspoon red pepper flakes**

SALAD

- **½ (14-ounce) can quartered artichoke hearts, drained**
- **5 ounces grape or cherry tomatoes, halved**
- **½ cup chopped green bell pepper**
- **¼ cup finely chopped red onion**
- **2 ounces mozzarella cheese, cut into ¼-inch cubes**

1 For dressing, whisk vinegar, oregano, sugar, salt and red pepper flakes in large bowl.

2 Add artichokes, tomatoes, bell pepper, onion and cheese to dressing; toss to coat. Serve immediately or refrigerate 1 hour to allow flavors to blend.

MAKES 4 SERVINGS

¾ CUP PER SERVING:

calories 90

total fat 3g

saturated fat 2g

sodium 420mg

carbs 12g

fiber 2g

sugar 3g

protein 5g

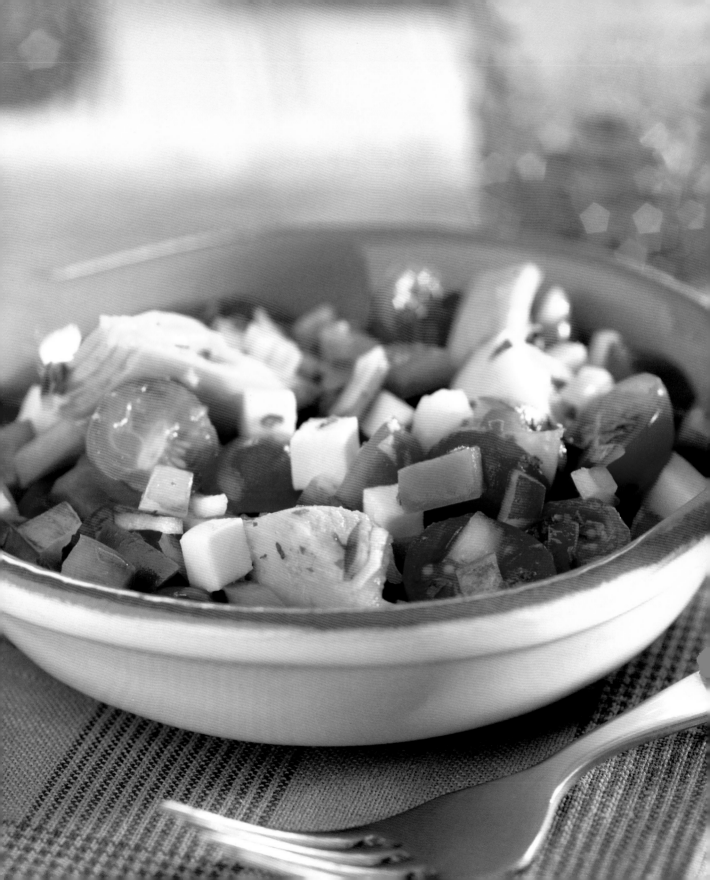

Roasted Brussels Sprouts Salad

BRUSSELS SPROUTS

- **1 pound brussels sprouts, trimmed and halved**
- **2 tablespoons olive oil**
- **½ teaspoon salt**

SALAD

- **2 cups coarsely chopped baby kale**
- **2 cups coarsely chopped romaine lettuce**
- **1½ cups candied pecans***
- **1 cup halved red grapes**
- **1 cup diced cucumber**
- **½ cup dried cranberries**
- **½ cup fresh blueberries**
- **½ cup chopped red onion**
- **¼ cup toasted pumpkin seeds (pepitas)**
- **1 container (4 ounces) crumbled goat cheese**

DRESSING

- **½ cup olive oil**
- **6 tablespoons balsamic vinegar**
- **6 tablespoons strawberry jam**
- **2 teaspoons Dijon mustard**
- **1 teaspoon salt**

Candied or glazed pecans may be found in the produce section of the supermarket with other salad toppings, or they may be found in the snack or baking aisles.

1 For brussels sprouts, preheat oven to 400°F. Spray large baking sheet with nonstick cooking spray.

2 Combine brussels sprouts, 2 tablespoons oil and ½ teaspoon salt in medium bowl; toss to coat. Arrange brussels sprouts in single layer, cut sides down, on prepared baking sheet. Roast 20 minutes or until tender and browned, stirring once halfway through roasting. Cool completely on baking sheet.

3 For salad, combine kale, lettuce, pecans, grapes, cucumber, cranberries, blueberries, onion and pumpkin seeds in large bowl. Top with brussels sprouts and cheese.

4 For dressing, whisk ½ cup oil, vinegar, jam, mustard and 1 teaspoon salt in small bowl until well blended. Pour dressing over salad; toss gently to coat.

MAKES 6 SERVINGS

1⅓ CUPS PER SERVING:

calories **600**

total fat **44g**

saturated fat **8g**

sodium **750mg**

carbs **54g**

fiber **6g**

sugar **41g**

protein **11g**

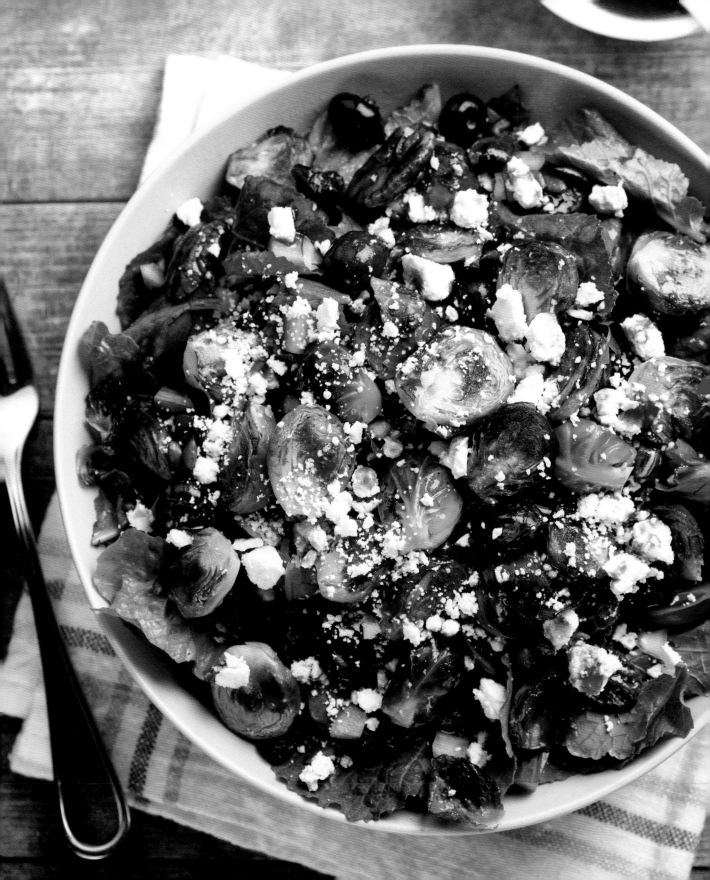

Chopped Italian Salad

10 cups chopped
    romaine lettuce

⅓ cup chopped red
    onion

20 slices reduced-fat
    turkey pepperoni,
    quartered

1 can (2¼ ounces)
    sliced black olives,
    rinsed and drained

1 can (about
    15 ounces)
    reduced-sodium
    chickpeas, rinsed
    and drained

⅓ cup light balsamic
    vinaigrette
    dressing

⅓ cup shredded
    Parmesan cheese

1 Combine lettuce, onion, pepperoni,
  olives and chickpeas in large bowl.

2 Add dressing; toss gently to coat.
  Sprinkle with cheese.

**MAKES
6 SERVINGS**

1 CUP
PER SERVING:

calories 180

total fat 8g

saturated
fat 2g

sodium
820mg

carbs 16g

fiber 4g

sugar 6g

protein 13g

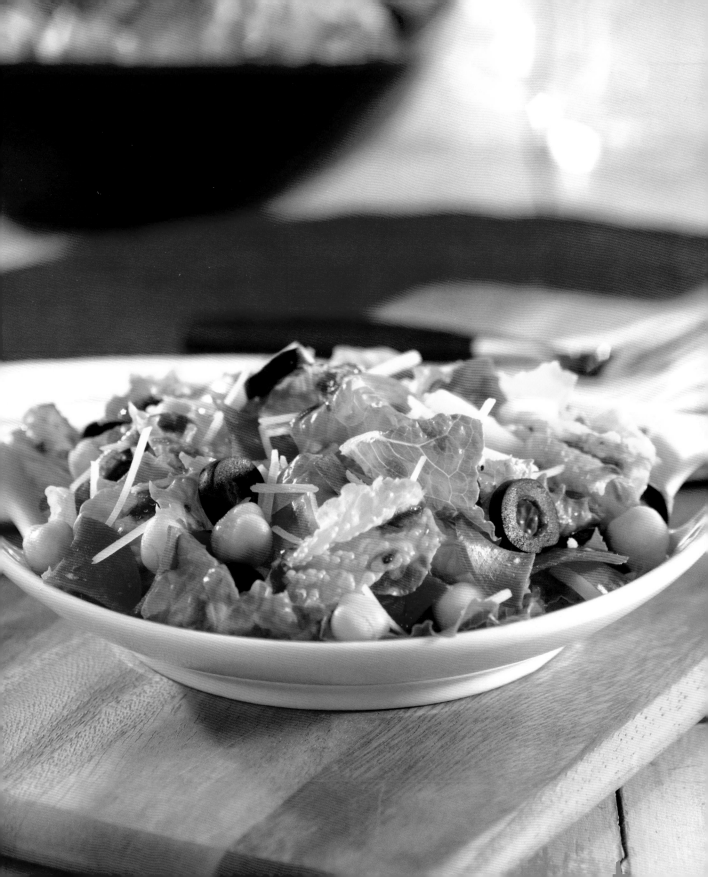

Spinach Salad

DRESSING

¼ **cup balsamic vinegar**

1 **clove garlic, minced**

½ **teaspoon sugar**

¼ **teaspoon salt**

⅛ **teaspoon black pepper**

¼ **cup olive oil**

¼ **cup vegetable oil**

SALAD

8 **cups packed baby spinach**

1 **cup diced tomatoes (about 2 medium)**

1 **cup drained mandarin oranges**

1 **cup glazed pecans***

½ **cup crumbled feta cheese**

½ **cup chopped red onion**

½ **cup dried cranberries**

1 **can (3 ounces) crispy rice noodles****

4 **teaspoons toasted sesame seeds**

Look for glazed pecans in the produce section of the supermarket with other salad toppings, the snack aisle or the baking aisle. Or make your own (see Tip).

**Crispy rice noodles can be found with canned chow mein noodles in the Asian section of the supermarket.*

1 For dressing, whisk vinegar, garlic, sugar, salt and pepper in medium bowl until blended. Slowly whisk in olive oil and vegetable oil in thin, steady stream until well blended.

2 For salad, divide spinach among six serving bowls. Top with tomatoes, mandarin oranges, pecans, cheese, onion and cranberries. Sprinkle with rice noodles and sesame seeds. Drizzle each salad with 3 tablespoons dressing.

TIP: To make glazed pecans, combine 1 cup pecan halves, ¼ cup sugar, 1 tablespoon butter and ½ teaspoon salt in medium skillet; cook and stir over medium heat 5 minutes or until sugar mixture is dark brown and nuts are well coated. Spread on large plate; cool completely. Break into pieces or coarsely chop.

MAKES 6 SERVINGS

⅙ OF TOTAL RECIPE PER SERVING:

calories **530**

total fat **38g**

saturated fat **5g**

sodium **460mg**

carbs **43g**

fiber **5g**

sugar **23g**

protein **8g**

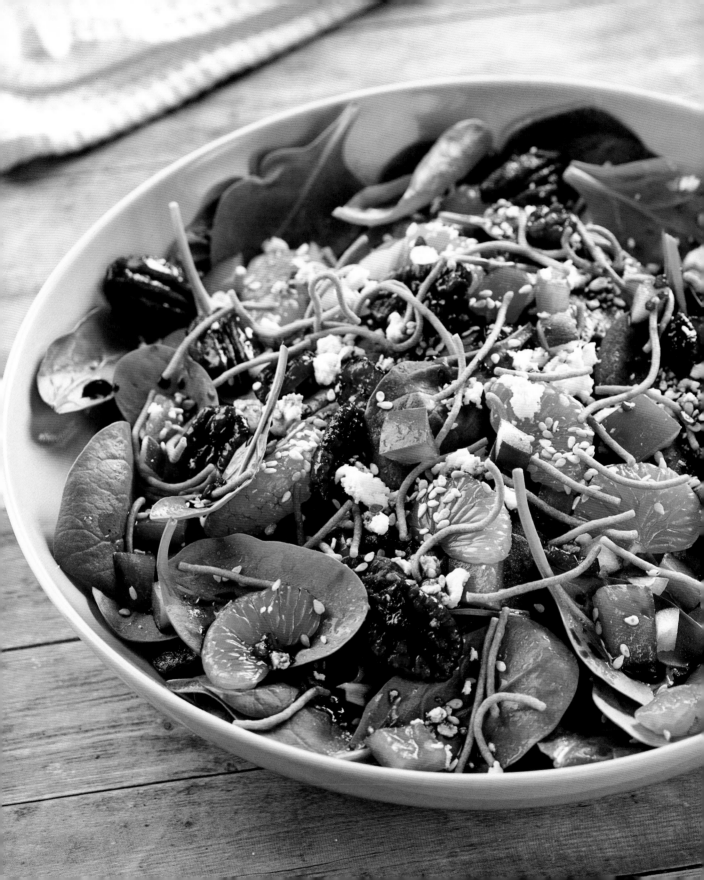

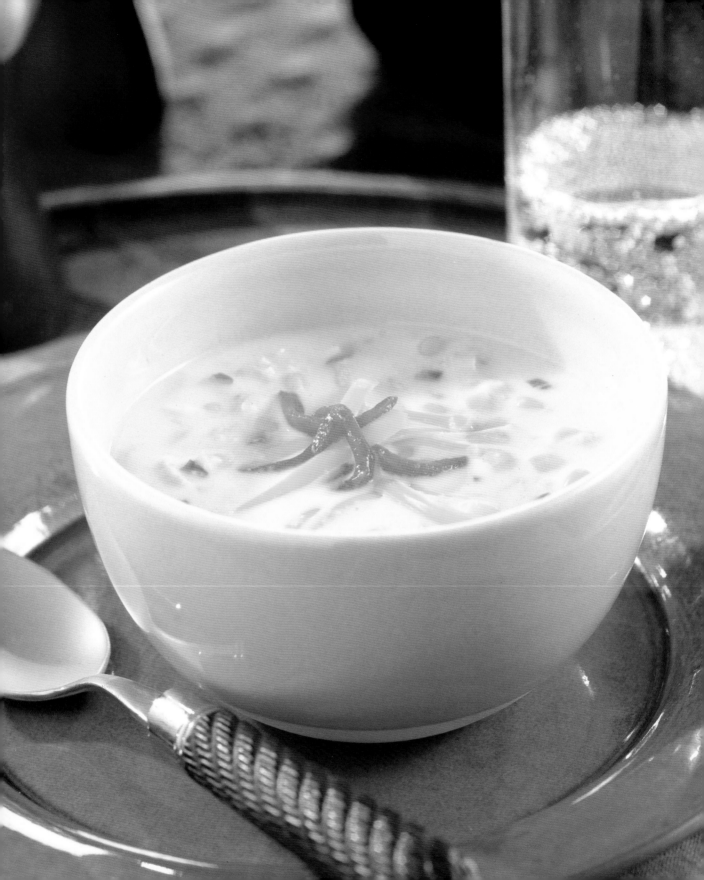

Corn and Jalapeño Chowder

4 cups thawed frozen corn, divided

2 cups reduced-sodium vegetable broth, divided

2 jalapeño peppers, seeded and finely chopped

¼ teaspoon onion salt*

1½ teaspoons whole cumin seeds, crushed

1 cup fat-free half-and-half

4 tablespoons (1 ounce) shredded reduced-fat Cheddar cheese

4 tablespoons thinly sliced roasted red pepper

Or substitute ⅛ teaspoon each salt and onion powder.

1 Place 2 cups corn and 1 cup broth in food processor; process until nearly smooth.

2 Combine corn mixture, remaining corn, remaining broth, jalapeños, onion salt and cumin seeds in large saucepan. Bring to a boil. Reduce heat to medium-low; cover and simmer 5 minutes.

3 Stir in half-and-half; cook and stir until heated through. Sprinkle each serving with 1 tablespoon cheese and 1 tablespoon roasted pepper.

MAKES 4 SERVINGS

½ CUP PER SERVING:

calories 200

total fat 4g

saturated fat 2g

sodium 380mg

carbs 36g

fiber 3g

sugar 8g

protein 9g

Turkey Albondigas Soup

¼ **cup uncooked brown rice**

MEATBALLS

½ **pound ground turkey**

1 **tablespoon minced onion**

1 **teaspoon chopped fresh cilantro**

1 **teaspoon fat-free (skim) milk**

½ **teaspoon hot pepper sauce**

⅛ **teaspoon dried oregano**

⅛ **teaspoon black pepper**

BROTH

1 **teaspoon olive oil**

2 **tablespoons chopped onion**

1 **clove garlic, minced**

2½ **cups reduced-sodium chicken broth**

2 **teaspoons hot pepper sauce**

1 **teaspoon tomato paste**

⅛ **teaspoon black pepper**

3 **small carrots, sliced into rounds (about 1 cup)**

½ **medium zucchini, quartered lengthwise and cut crosswise into ½-inch slices**

½ **medium yellow crookneck squash, quartered lengthwise and cut crosswise into ½-inch slices**

Lime wedges (optional)

1 Prepare rice according to package directions.

2 Meanwhile, combine turkey, minced onion, cilantro, milk, ½ teaspoon hot pepper sauce, oregano and ⅛ teaspoon black pepper in medium bowl. Mix lightly until blended. Shape mixture into 1-inch balls.

3 For broth, heat oil in large saucepan over medium heat. Add chopped onion and garlic; cook and stir until golden brown. Add broth, 2 teaspoons hot pepper sauce, tomato paste and ⅛ teaspoon black pepper; bring to a boil over high heat.

4 Reduce heat to low. Add meatballs and carrots to broth; simmer 15 minutes. Add zucchini, squash and cooked rice; simmer 5 to 10 minutes or just until vegetables are tender.

5 Ladle into bowls; garnish with lime wedges.

MAKES 2 SERVINGS

½ OF TOTAL RECIPE PER SERVING:

calories 280

total fat 5g

saturated fat 1g

sodium 870mg

carbs 31g

fiber 4g

sugar 8g

protein 31g

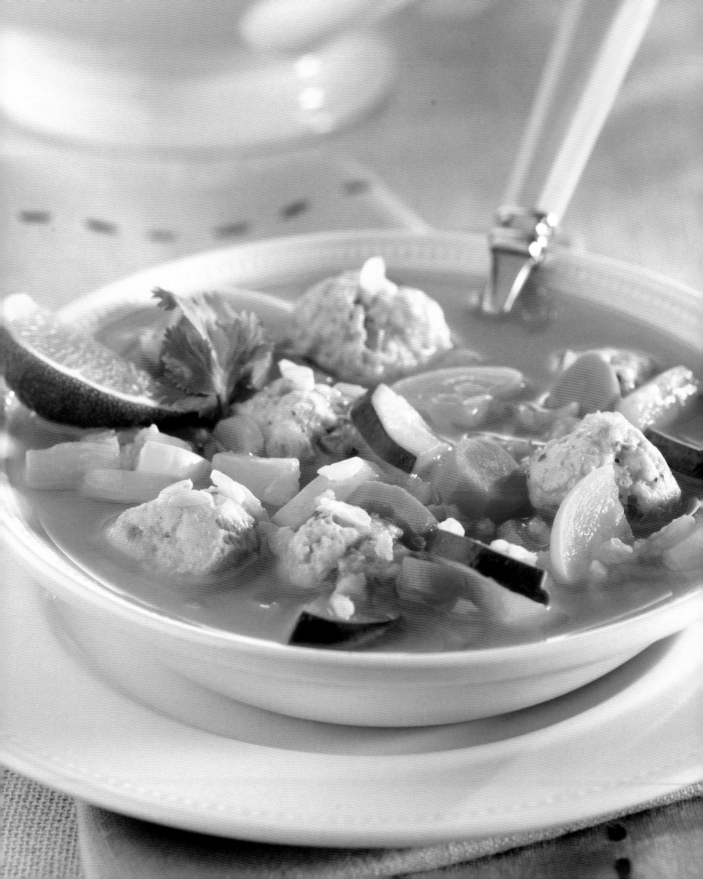

Rustic Vegetable Soup

1 to 2 baking potatoes, cut into ½-inch pieces

1 bag (10 ounces) frozen mixed vegetables, thawed

1 bag (10 ounces) frozen cut green beans, thawed

1 medium green bell pepper, chopped

1 jar (16 ounces) picante sauce

1 can (about 10 ounces) condensed beef broth, undiluted

½ teaspoon sugar

¼ cup finely chopped fresh parsley

SLOW COOKER DIRECTIONS

1 Combine potatoes, mixed vegetables, green beans, bell pepper, picante sauce, broth and sugar in slow cooker.

2 Cover; cook on LOW 8 hours or on HIGH 4 hours. Stir in parsley just before serving.

NOTE: To make this easy soup on the stove top, combine all the ingredients except for the parsley in a large saucepan. Simmer, covered, over medium heat until the potatoes are tender and the flavors are blended.

MAKES 8 SERVINGS

⅛ OF TOTAL RECIPE PER SERVING:

calories 160
total fat 0g
saturated fat 0g
sodium 1080mg
carbs 32g
fiber 8g
sugar 6g
protein 6g

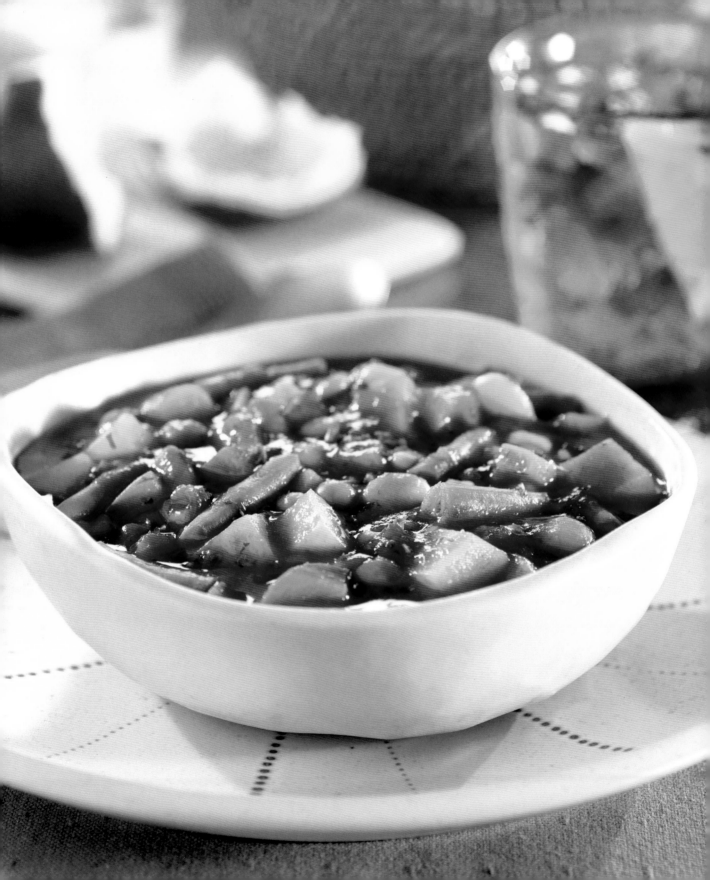

Chicken Rotini Soup

2 tablespoons butter

½ pound boneless skinless chicken breasts, cut into ½-inch pieces

½ medium onion, chopped

4 ounces mushrooms, sliced

4 cups reduced-sodium chicken broth

1 teaspoon Worcestershire sauce

¼ teaspoon dried tarragon

¾ cup uncooked rotini pasta

1 small zucchini

1 Melt butter in Dutch oven or large saucepan over medium heat. Add chicken, onion and mushrooms; cook and stir 5 minutes or until onion is softened. Stir in broth, Worcestershire sauce and tarragon. Bring to a boil over high heat. Stir in pasta. Reduce heat to medium-low; simmer, uncovered, 5 minutes.

2 Cut zucchini into ⅛-inch slices; halve any large slices. Add to soup; simmer, uncovered, about 5 minutes or until pasta is tender.

MAKES 4 SERVINGS

¼ OF TOTAL RECIPE PER SERVING:

calories 220

total fat 8g

saturated fat 4g

sodium 600mg

carbs 18g

fiber 1g

sugar 3g

protein 20g

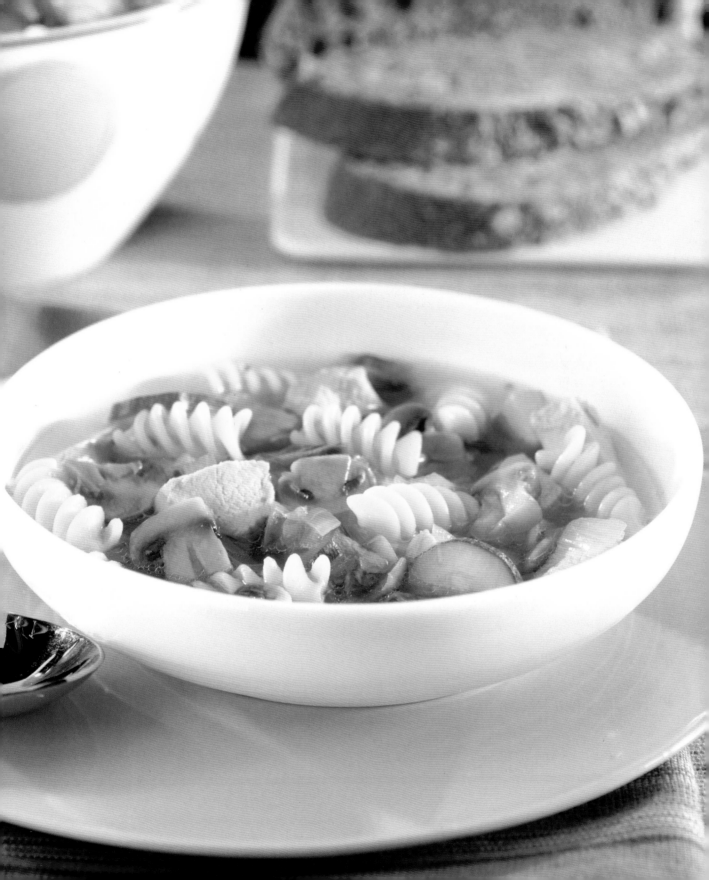

Seafood Stew

2 tablespoons butter

1 cup chopped onion

1 cup green bell pepper strips

1 teaspoon dried dill
Dash ground red pepper

1 can (about 14 ounces) diced tomatoes

½ cup dry white wine

2 tablespoons lime juice

8 ounces swordfish steak, cut into 1-inch cubes

8 ounces bay or sea scallops, cut into quarters

1 bottle (8 ounces) clam juice

2 tablespoons cornstarch

2 cups frozen diced potatoes, thawed and drained

8 ounces frozen cooked medium shrimp, thawed and drained

½ cup whipping cream
Salt and black pepper

1 Melt butter in Dutch oven over medium-high heat. Add onion, bell pepper, dill and ground red pepper; cook and stir 5 minutes or until vegetables are tender.

2 Reduce heat to medium. Add tomatoes, wine and lime juice; bring to a boil. Add swordfish and scallops; cook and stir 2 minutes.

3 Stir clam juice into cornstarch in small bowl until smooth.

4 Increase heat to high. Add potatoes, shrimp, cream and clam juice mixture; bring to a boil. Remove from heat; season to taste with salt and black pepper.

MAKES 6 SERVINGS

¹/₆ OF TOTAL RECIPE PER SERVING:

calories 290

total fat 14g

saturated fat 8g

sodium 760g

carbs 20g

fiber 3g

sugar 5g

protein 19g

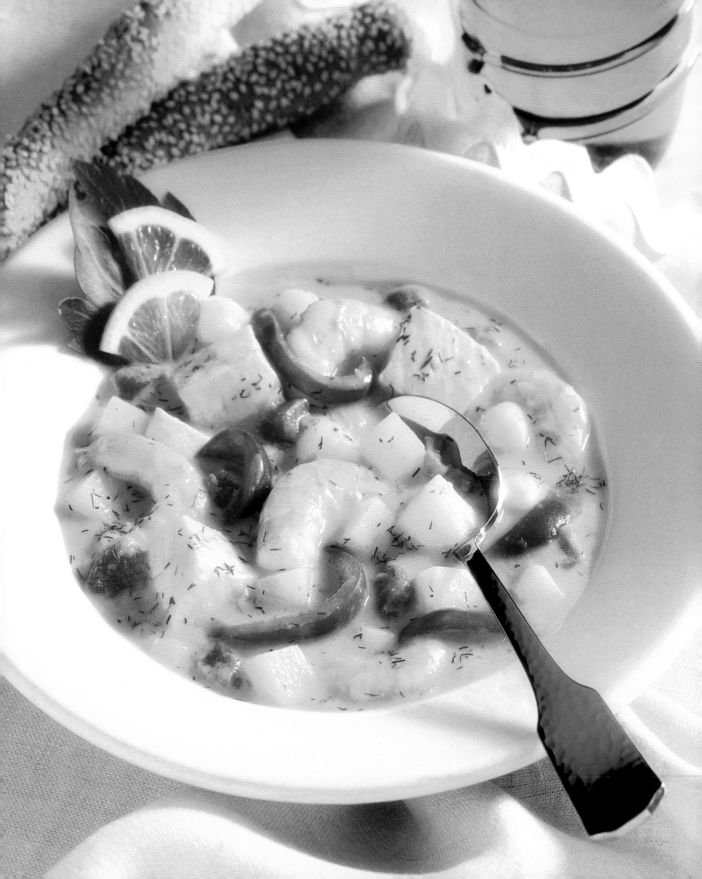

Chickpea-Vegetable Soup

1 teaspoon olive oil

1 cup chopped onion

½ cup chopped green bell pepper

2 cloves garlic, minced

2 cans (about 14 ounces each) diced tomatoes

3 cups water

2 cups broccoli florets

1 can (about 15 ounces) chickpeas, rinsed, drained and slightly mashed

½ cup (3 ounces) uncooked orzo or rosamarina pasta

1 bay leaf

1 tablespoon chopped fresh thyme or 1 teaspoon dried thyme

1 tablespoon chopped fresh rosemary or 1 teaspoon dried rosemary

1 tablespoon lime or lemon juice

½ teaspoon ground turmeric

¼ teaspoon salt

¼ teaspoon ground red pepper

¼ cup pepitas (pumpkin seeds) or sunflower kernels

1 Heat oil in large saucepan over medium heat. Add onion, bell pepper and garlic; cook and stir 5 minutes or until vegetables are softened.

2 Add tomatoes, water, broccoli, chickpeas, orzo, bay leaf, thyme, rosemary, lime juice, turmeric, salt and ground red pepper. Bring to a boil over high heat. Reduce heat to medium-low; cover and simmer 10 to 12 minutes or until orzo is tender.

3 Remove and discard bay leaf. Ladle soup into bowls; sprinkle with pepitas.

MAKES 4 SERVINGS

¼ OF TOTAL RECIPE PER SERVING:

calories 300

total fat 6g

saturated fat 1g

sodium 280mg

carbs 48g

fiber 9g

sugar 0g

protein 13g

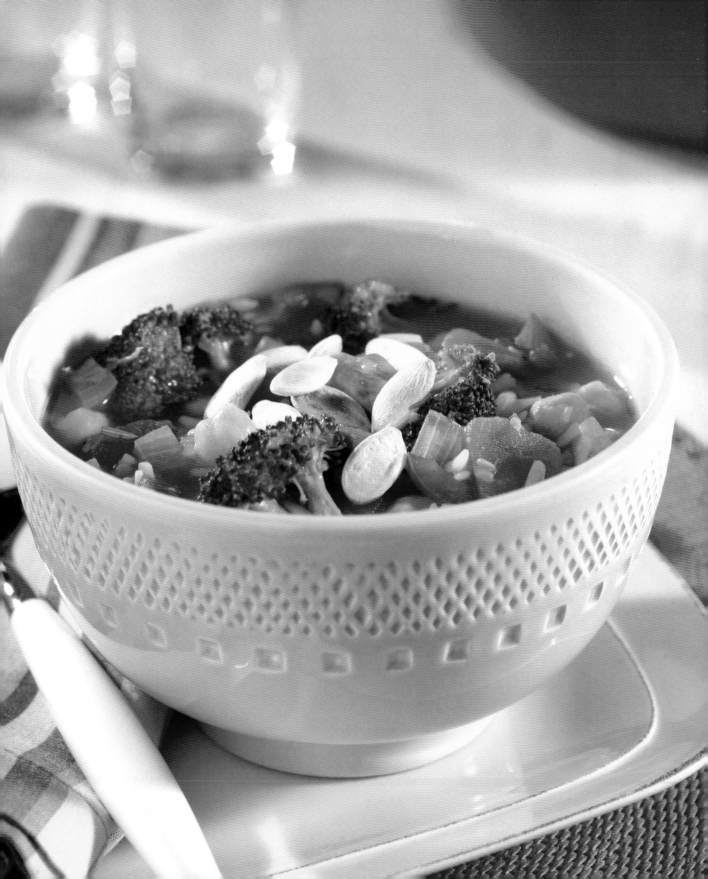

Italian-Style Bean Soup

1½ cups dried Great
   Northern or navy
   beans, rinsed and
   sorted

4 cups vegetable
   broth

1 cup water

1 cup pasta sauce

1 tablespoon dried
   minced onion

2 teaspoons dried
   basil

1 teaspoon dried
   parsley flakes

½ teaspoon minced
   fresh garlic

1½ cups uncooked
   medium pasta
   shells

8 ounces fresh baby
   spinach (optional)

   Salt and black
   pepper

¼ cup grated
   Parmesan cheese

1 Place beans in large bowl; cover with water. Soak 6 to 8 hours or overnight.

2 Drain beans; discard water. Combine soaked beans, broth, 1 cup water, pasta sauce, onion, basil, parsley flakes and garlic in Dutch oven; bring to a boil over high heat. Reduce heat to low; cover and simmer 2 to 2½ hours.

3 Add pasta; cover and simmer 15 to 20 minutes or until pasta and beans are tender. Stir in spinach, if desired; let stand until wilted. Season to taste with salt and pepper. Ladle into bowls; top with cheese.

TIP: To quick soak beans, place in large saucepan; cover with water. Bring to a boil over high heat; boil 2 minutes. Remove from heat; let soak, covered, 1 hour. Skip step 1 and proceed with step 2.

**MAKES
8 SERVINGS**

⅛ OF TOTAL RECIPE
PER SERVING:

calories 220

total fat 3g

saturated
fat 1g

sodium
370g

carbs 38g

fiber 6g

sugar 3g

protein 12g

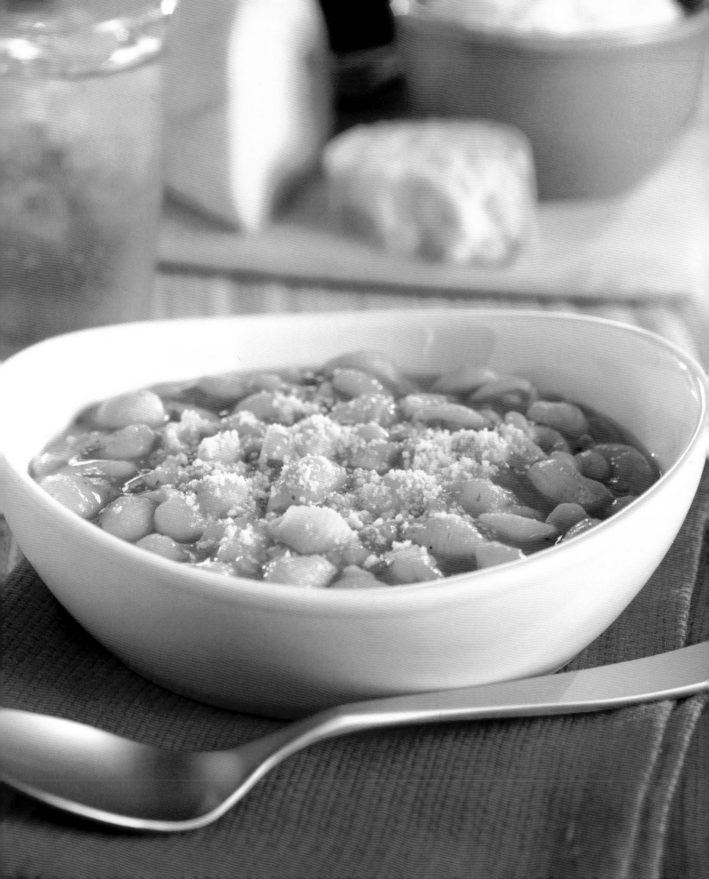

One-Pot Chinese Chicken Soup

6 cups reduced-sodium chicken broth

2 cups water

1 pound boneless skinless chicken thighs

⅓ cup reduced-sodium soy sauce

1 package (16 ounces) frozen stir-fry vegetables

6 ounces uncooked dried thin Chinese egg noodles

1 to 3 tablespoons sriracha sauce

1 Combine broth, water, chicken and soy sauce in medium saucepan; bring to a boil over high heat. Reduce heat to low; cover and simmer 20 minutes or until chicken is cooked through and very tender. Remove chicken to bowl; let stand until cool enough to handle.

2 Meanwhile, add vegetables and noodles to broth in saucepan; bring to a boil over high heat. Reduce heat to medium-high; cook 5 minutes or until noodles are tender and vegetables are heated through.

3 Shred chicken into bite-size pieces. Stir chicken and 1 tablespoon sriracha into soup; taste and add additional sriracha for a spicier flavor.

MAKES 6 SERVINGS

⅙ OF TOTAL RECIPE PER SERVING:

calories 250

total fat 4g

saturated fat 1g

sodium 1210mg

carbs 26g

fiber 0g

sugar 5g

protein 24g

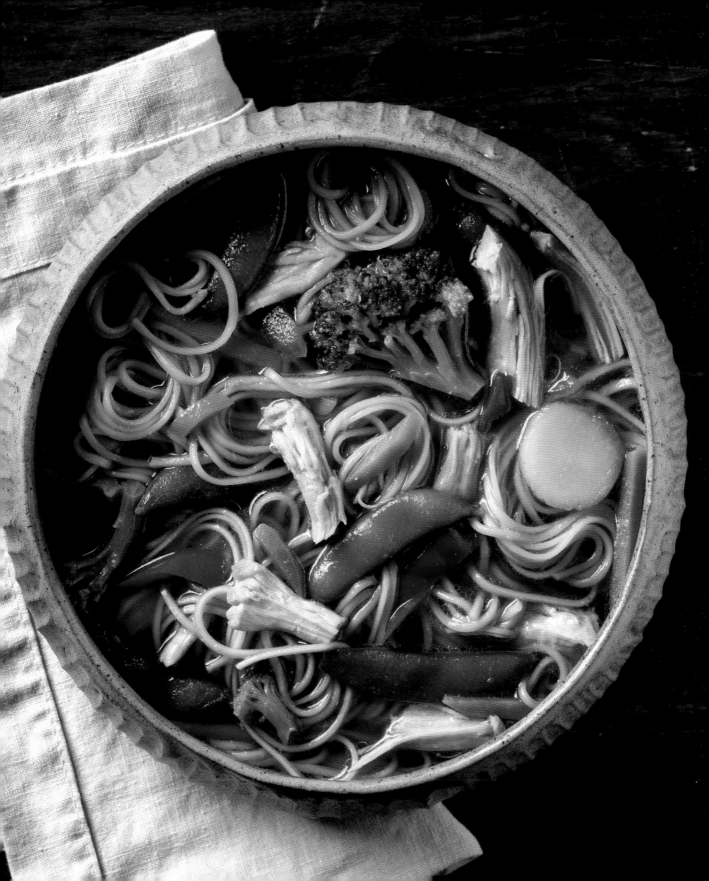

Curry Red Lentil and Chickpea Stew

- 1 tablespoon olive oil
- 1 onion, chopped
- 3 cloves garlic, minced
- 2 tablespoons minced fresh ginger
- 1 tablespoon curry powder
- 2 teaspoons ground turmeric
- ⅛ teaspoon ground red pepper
- 4 cups vegetable broth
- 1¼ cups uncooked red lentils (8 ounces)
- 1 can (about 15 ounces) chickpeas, rinsed and drained
- 1 can (about 13 ounces) coconut milk
- 1 package (5 ounces) baby spinach
- Salt
- Chopped fresh parsley and/or shredded coconut (optional)

1 Heat oil in large saucepan over medium-high heat. Add onion; cook and stir 5 minutes or until softened. Add garlic, ginger, curry powder, turmeric and ground red pepper; cook and stir 1 minute. Add broth; bring to a boil. Stir in lentils; cook 15 minutes, stirring frequently.

2 Stir in chickpeas and coconut milk; cook 5 to 10 minutes or until lentils are tender, chickpeas are heated through and stew is slightly thickened. Stir in spinach; cook and stir 2 to 3 minutes or just until spinach is wilted. Season to taste with salt.

3 Ladle into bowls; garnish with parsley and/or coconut.

MAKES 6 SERVINGS

ABOUT 1 CUP PER SERVING:

calories 380
total fat 18g
saturated fat 13g
sodium 640mg
carbs 41g
fiber 14g
sugar 3g
protein 15g

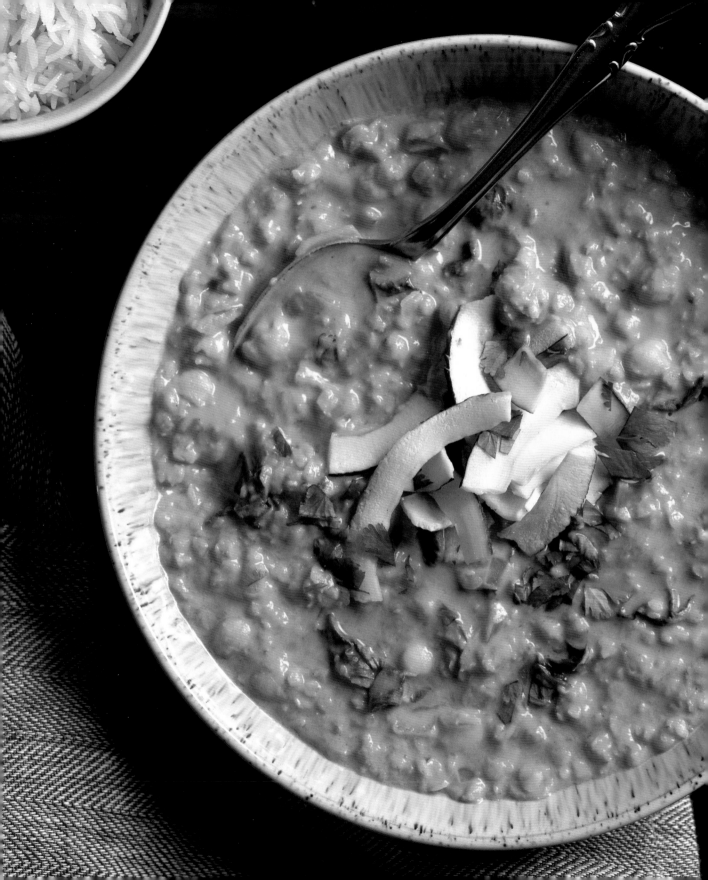

Peppery Sicilian Chicken Soup

MAKES
10 SERVINGS

$1/_{10}$ OF TOTAL RECIPE
PER SERVING:

calories 300

total fat 6g

saturated
fat 1g

sodium
890mg

carbs 32g

fiber 4g

sugar 5g

protein 29g

2 tablespoons olive
   oil

1 medium onion,
   chopped

1 green bell pepper,
   chopped

3 stalks celery,
   chopped

3 carrots, chopped

3 cloves garlic,
   minced

3 containers
   (32 ounces each)
   reduced-sodium
   chicken broth

2 pounds boneless
   skinless chicken
   breasts

1 can (28 ounces)
   diced tomatoes

2 baking potatoes,
   peeled and cut
   into ¼-inch pieces

1½ teaspoons ground
   white pepper*

1½ teaspoons ground
   black pepper

½ cup chopped fresh
   parsley

8 ounces uncooked
   ditalini pasta

   Salt

   *Or substitute
   additional black pepper
   for the white pepper.

1 Heat oil in large saucepan or Dutch oven over medium heat. Stir in onion, bell pepper, celery and carrots. Reduce heat to medium-low; cover and cook 10 to 15 minutes or until vegetables are tender but not browned, stirring occasionally. Stir in garlic; cover and cook 5 minutes.

2 Stir in broth, chicken, tomatoes, potatoes, white pepper and black pepper; bring to a boil. Reduce heat to low; cover and simmer 1 hour. Remove chicken to plate; set aside until cool enough to handle. Shred chicken and return to saucepan with parsley.

3 Meanwhile, cook pasta in medium saucepan of salted boiling water 7 minutes (or 1 minute less than package directs for al dente). Drain pasta and add to soup. Season to taste with salt.

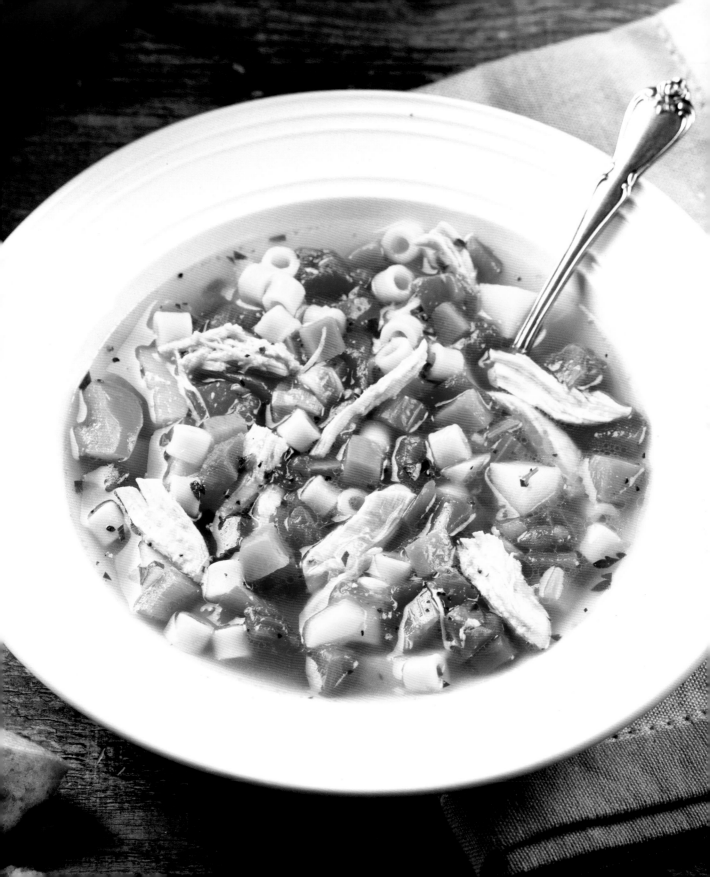

Turkey Vegetable Rice Soup

1½ pounds turkey
   drumsticks
   (2 small)

8 cups water

1 medium onion, cut
   into quarters

2 tablespoons soy
   sauce

¼ teaspoon black
   pepper

1 bay leaf

2 carrots, sliced

⅓ cup uncooked rice

4 ounces mushrooms,
   sliced

1 cup fresh snow
   peas, cut in half
   crosswise

1 cup coarsely
   chopped bok choy

1 Place turkey in large saucepan or Dutch
   oven. Add water, onion, soy sauce,
   pepper and bay leaf; bring to a boil over
   high heat. Reduce heat to medium-low;
   simmer, uncovered, 1½ hours or until
   turkey is tender.

2 Remove turkey to plate; set aside until
   cool enough to handle. Let broth cool
   slightly; skim fat. Remove and discard
   bay leaf. Remove turkey meat from
   bones; discard skin and bones. Cut
   turkey into bite-size pieces.

3 Add carrots and rice to broth in
   saucepan; bring to a boil over high
   heat. Reduce heat to medium-low;
   cook 10 minutes.

4 Add mushrooms and turkey to soup;
   bring to a boil over high heat. Reduce
   heat to medium-low; cook 5 minutes.
   Add snow peas and bok choy; bring to
   a boil over high heat. Reduce heat to
   medium-low; cook 8 minutes or until rice
   and vegetables are tender.

**MAKES
6 SERVINGS**

⅙ OF TOTAL RECIPE
PER SERVING:

calories 240

total fat 8g

saturated
fat 3g

sodium
490mg

carbs 15g

fiber 2g

sugar 3g

protein 25g

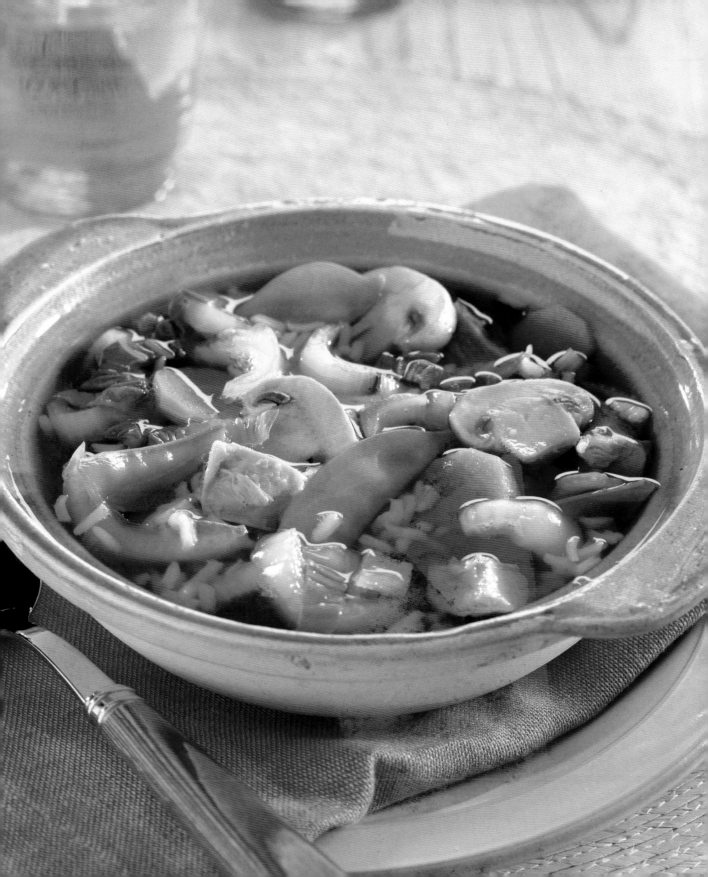

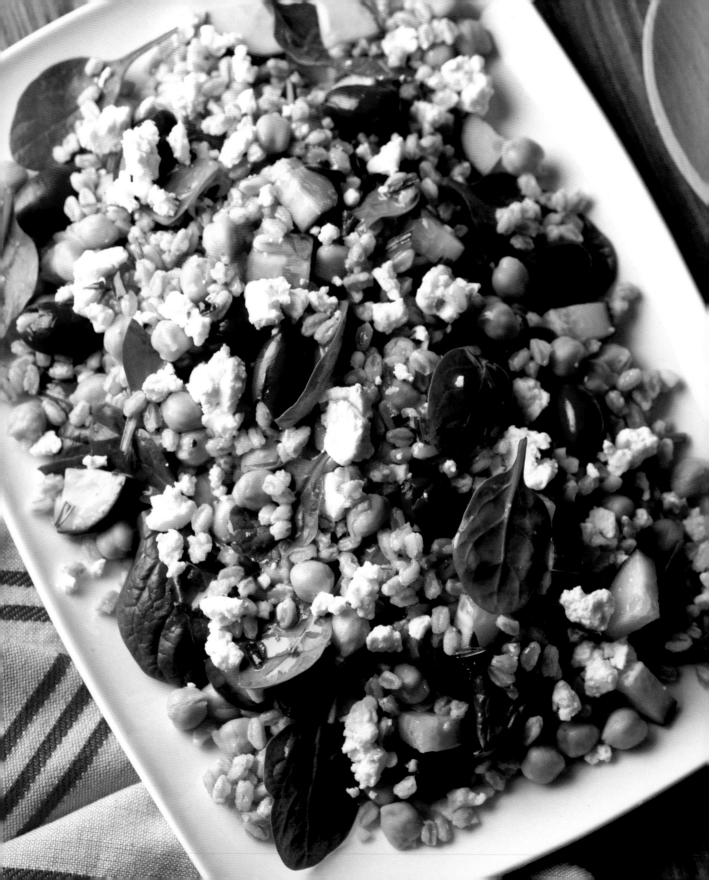

PASTA & GRAINS

Farro, Chickpea and Spinach Salad

- 1 cup uncooked pearled farro
- 3 cups baby spinach, stemmed
- 1 medium cucumber, chopped
- 1 can (about 15 ounces) chickpeas, rinsed and drained
- ¾ cup pitted kalamata olives
- ¼ cup olive oil
- 3 tablespoons white or golden balsamic vinegar*
- 1 teaspoon chopped fresh rosemary *or* ½ teaspoon dried rosemary
- 1 clove garlic, minced
- 1 teaspoon salt
- ½ cup crumbled goat or feta cheese

Or stir ½ teaspoon sugar into 3 tablespoons cider vinegar.

1 Bring 4 cups water to a boil in medium saucepan; stir in farro. Reduce heat to medium-low; simmer 20 to 25 minutes or until farro is tender. Drain and rinse under cold water until cool.

2 Meanwhile, combine spinach, cucumber, chickpeas, olives, oil, vinegar, rosemary, garlic and salt in large bowl. Stir in farro until well blended. Add cheese; stir gently.

Turkey Sausage and Spinach Stuffed Shells

18 uncooked jumbo shell pasta

1 teaspoon olive oil

8 ounces Italian turkey sausage, casings removed

½ cup chopped onion

2 cloves garlic, minced

1 package (6 ounces) baby spinach

1 cup fat-free ricotta cheese

1½ cups tomato-basil pasta sauce, divided

½ cup grated Parmesan cheese, divided

¼ cup chopped fresh basil

1 Preheat oven to 375°F. Cook pasta in large saucepan of salted boiling water according to package directions for al dente; drain.

2 Meanwhile, heat oil in large nonstick skillet over medium heat. Add sausage, onion and garlic; cook 5 minutes or until sausage begins to brown, stirring to break up meat. Add spinach in batches; cook and stir until wilted. Remove from heat; stir in ricotta, ½ cup pasta sauce and ¼ cup Parmesan.

3 Fill shells evenly with turkey mixture. Arrange shells in 2-quart casserole. Spoon remaining 1 cup pasta sauce evenly over shells. Cover with foil.

4 Bake 30 to 35 minutes or until heated through. Top with remaining ¼ cup Parmesan and basil.

MAKES 6 SERVINGS

3 FILLED SHELLS PER SERVING:

calories 255

total fat 5g

saturated fat 2g

sodium 580mg

carbs 36g

fiber 4g

sugar 10g

protein 15g

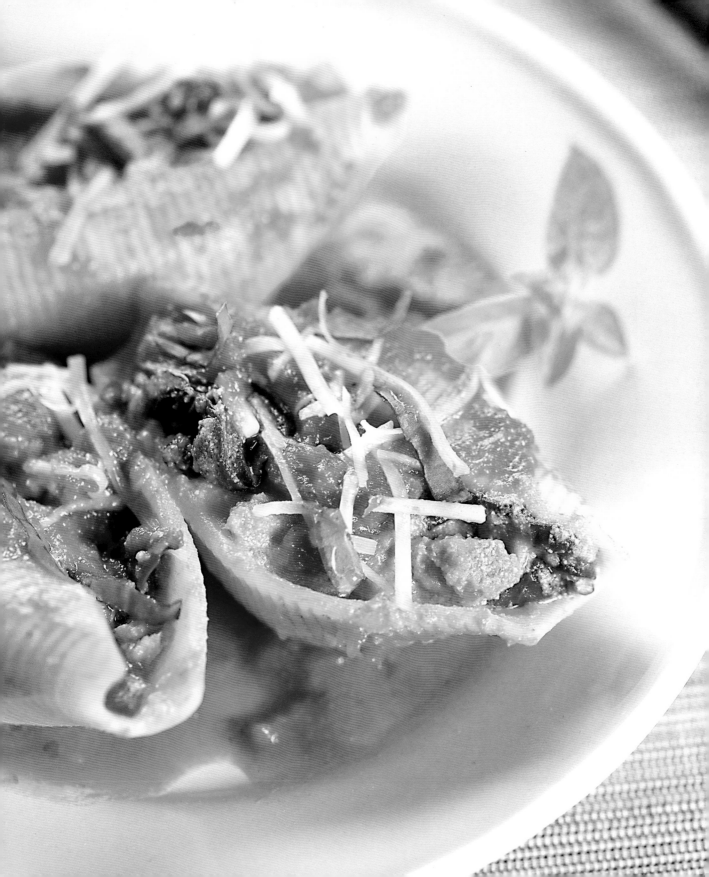

Three-Cheese Macaroni and Quinoa

6 ounces uncooked whole grain elbow macaroni (1½ cups)

½ cup uncooked quinoa

4 tablespoons (½ stick) butter, divided

½ cup panko

2 tablespoons all-purpose flour

½ teaspoon salt

1 cup milk

1 cup (4 ounces) shredded sharp Cheddar cheese

1 cup (4 ounces) shredded Monterey Jack cheese

¼ cup grated Parmesan cheese

1 Bring large saucepan of salted water to a boil over high heat. Stir in macaroni and quinoa; cook 10 minutes or until pasta and quinoa are al dente. Drain in fine-mesh strainer; place in large bowl.

2 Meanwhile, melt 2 tablespoons butter in medium saucepan over medium heat. Add panko; cook and stir 1 to 2 minutes or until golden. Transfer to small bowl.

3 Melt remaining 2 tablespoons butter in same saucepan over medium heat. Whisk in flour and salt; cook 1 minute without browning. Gradually whisk in milk; cook 5 minutes or until very thick. Stir in Cheddar and Monterey Jack until melted. Pour over macaroni mixture.

4 Scoop into bowls; top with Parmesan and toasted panko.

MAKES 4 SERVINGS

1½ CUPS PER SERVING:

calories 670

total fat 34g

saturated fat 20g

sodium 1110mg

carbs 63g

fiber 2g

sugar 5g

protein 29g

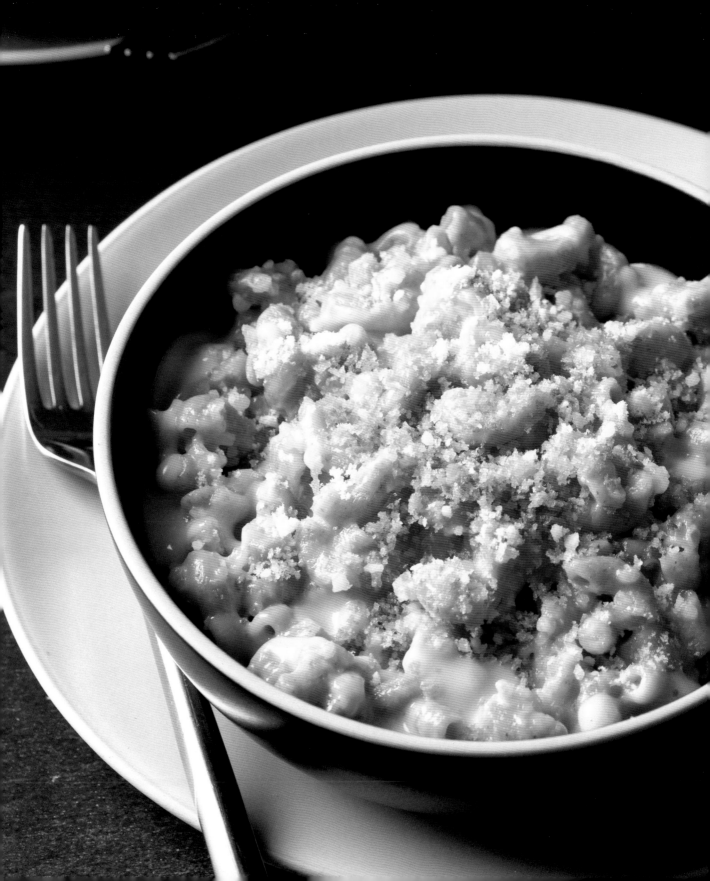

Herbed Vegetable Kasha

1 egg

1 cup kasha*

1 tablespoon olive oil

1 cup chopped broccoli

1 cup chopped red bell pepper

½ cup sliced cremini mushrooms

½ cup chopped onion

2 cloves garlic, minced

½ teaspoon dried dill

½ teaspoon dried rosemary

½ teaspoon dried thyme

½ teaspoon salt

¼ teaspoon black pepper

1 cup mushroom or vegetable broth

Kasha, or buckwheat groats, is buckwheat that has been toasted. It is commonly found in the Kosher section of the supermarket.

1 Beat egg in medium bowl; add kasha and mix until coated.

2 Heat large nonstick skillet over medium heat. Add kasha mixture; cook and stir 2 to 3 minutes or until kasha is dry and grains are separated. Transfer to large bowl; set aside.

3 Heat oil in same skillet over medium heat. Add broccoli, bell pepper, mushrooms, onion and garlic; cook and stir 5 to 7 minutes or until vegetables are crisp-tender. Add dill, rosemary, thyme, salt and black pepper; cook and stir 1 minute.

4 Add broth to skillet; bring to a boil. Stir in kasha. Reduce heat to medium-low; cover and cook 10 to 12 minutes or until liquid is absorbed and kasha is tender. Remove from heat; cover and let stand 5 minutes. Fluff with fork.

MAKES 4 SERVINGS

¼ OF TOTAL RECIPE PER SERVING:

calories 220

total fat 6g

saturated fat 0g

sodium 440mg

carbs 38g

fiber 6g

sugar 2g

protein 8g

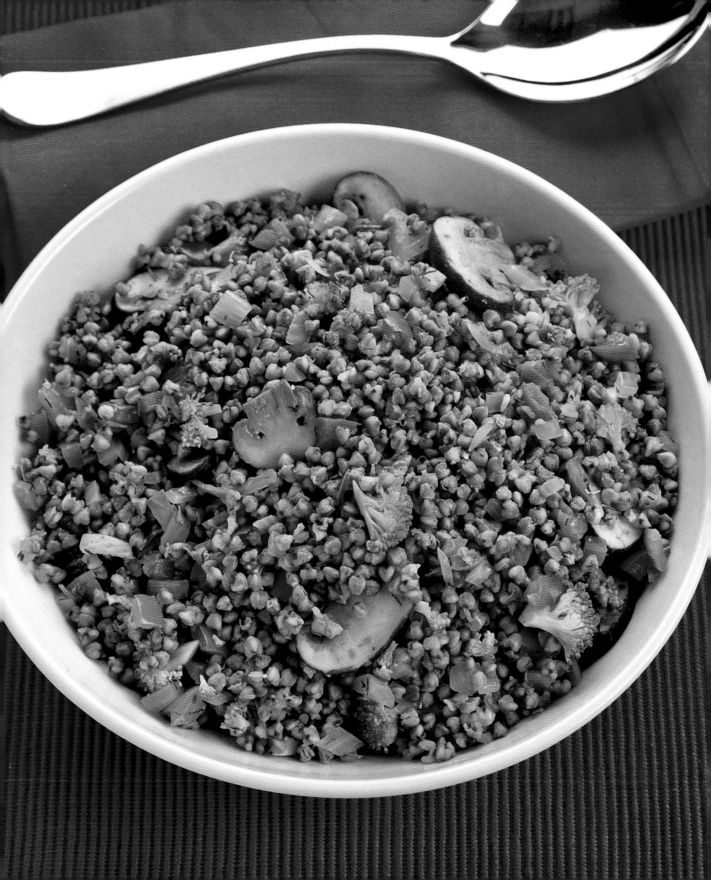

Tortellini with Artichokes, Olives and Feta Cheese

- 2 **packages (9 ounces each) refrigerated cheese-filled spinach tortellini**
- 2 **jars (4 ounces each) marinated artichoke heart quarters, drained***
- ½ **cup sliced pitted black olives**
- 2 **medium carrots, diagonally sliced**
- ½ **cup crumbled feta cheese**
- ½ **cup garlic Parmesan Italian salad dressing**

  Black pepper

  For additional flavor, add some artichoke marinade to tortellini with salad dressing.

1 Cook pasta in large saucepan of salted boiling water according to package directions. Drain in colander and rinse under cold water until cool.

2 Combine pasta, artichoke hearts, olives, carrots and cheese in large bowl. Add salad dressing; stir to coat. Season to taste with pepper.

MAKES 6 SERVINGS

⅙ OF TOTAL RECIPE PER SERVING:

calories 390

total fat 16g

saturated fat 5g

sodium 990mg

carbs 49g

fiber 2g

sugar 5g

protein 15g

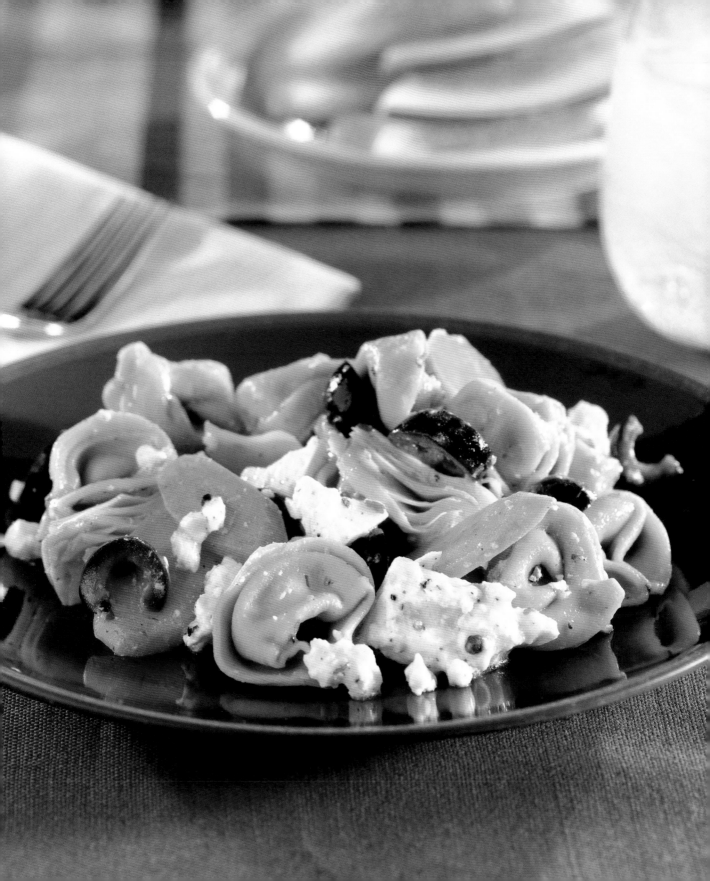

Barley and Mushroom Pilaf

- 2 cups reduced-sodium vegetable broth
- 1 cup quick cooking barley
- 4 teaspoons olive oil, divided
- 2 cups chopped onions
- 8 ounces sliced mushrooms
- 2 cloves garlic, minced
- 1 teaspoon dried oregano
- ½ teaspoon salt
- ¼ teaspoon black pepper
- Chopped fresh parsley

1 Bring broth to a boil in medium saucepan over high heat. Stir in barley. Reduce heat to low; cover and simmer 10 minutes.

2 Meanwhile, heat 1 teaspoon oil in large skillet over medium-high heat. Add onions; cook and stir 5 minutes or until softened. Add mushrooms, garlic and oregano; cook 4 minutes or until mushrooms begin to brown, stirring frequently.

3 Stir vegetables, remaining 3 teaspoons oil, salt and pepper into barley. Sprinkle with parsley; serve immediately.

MAKES 4 SERVINGS

½ CUP PER SERVING:

calories 140
total fat 3g
saturated fat 0g
sodium 250mg
carbs 25g
fiber 5g
sugar 3g
protein 4g

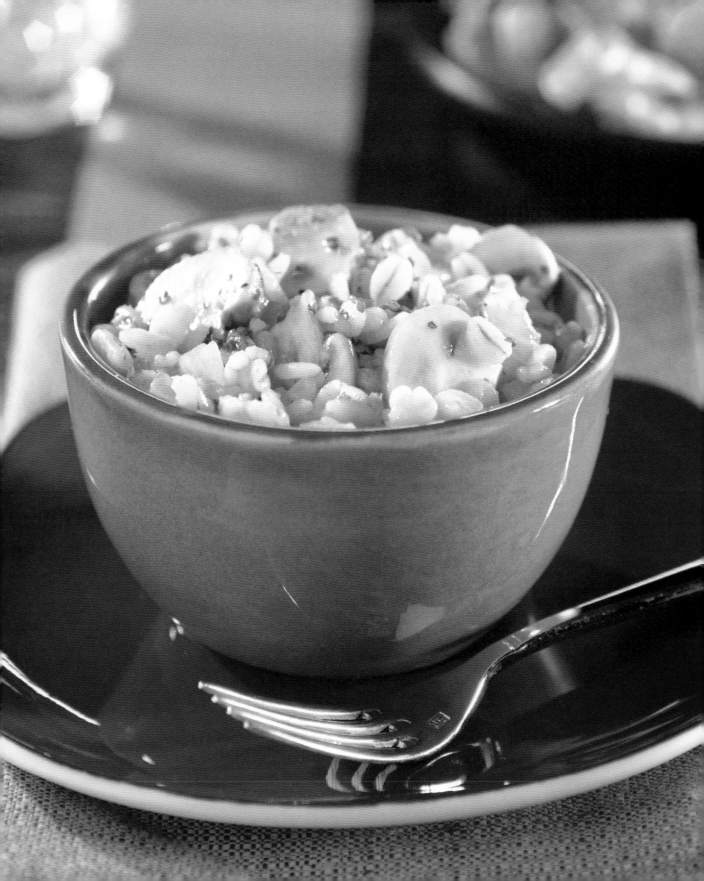

Spaghetti with Creamy Tomato-Pepper Sauce

- 1 package (16 ounces) uncooked whole grain or whole wheat spaghetti
- 2 tablespoons olive oil
- 1 small onion, chopped
- 2 tablespoons minced garlic
- 1 large red bell pepper, chopped
- 2 large tomatoes, seeded and chopped (about 3 cups)
- ½ cup grated Parmesan cheese
- ¼ cup fat-free half-and-half
- ½ teaspoon black pepper

1 Cook pasta in large saucepan of salted boiling water according to package directions for al dente. Drain and return to saucepan; keep warm.

2 Meanwhile, heat oil in large skillet over medium heat. Add onion and garlic; cook and stir 5 minutes or until onion is softened. Add bell pepper; cook 4 minutes or until pepper is crisp-tender. Stir in tomatoes.

3 Remove from heat; let stand 2 minutes to cool slightly. Return skillet to low heat. Gradually stir in cheese, half-and-half and black pepper; cook 5 minutes or until heated through, stirring frequently. Pour over pasta; mix well.

NOTE: To seed a tomato, cut it in half side-to-side, not top to bottom. Then, scrape the seeds out using a teaspoon. If you want to make a tomato cup, also remove the "walls" between the seed compartments, using the teaspoon to scrape them away.

MAKES 6 SERVINGS

1¼ CUPS PER SERVING:

calories 350

total fat 11g

saturated fat 3g

sodium 170mg

carbs 52g

fiber 8g

sugar 5g

protein 14g

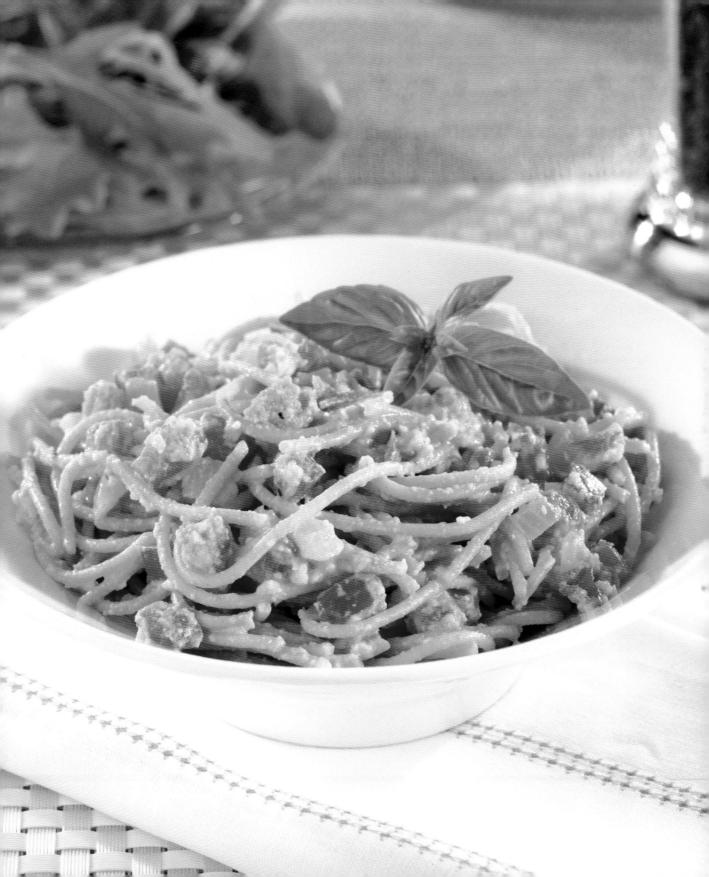

Rotini Pasta Salad with Chicken

⅓ cup plus
    3 tablespoons
    olive oil, divided

1 teaspoon salt

1 teaspoon dried
    oregano

1 teaspoon paprika

¼ teaspoon black
    pepper

2 cloves garlic,
    minced, divided

4 boneless skinless
    chicken breasts
    (4 to 6 ounces
    each)

8 ounces uncooked
    rotini pasta

1 cup grape
    tomatoes, halved

½ seedless cucumber,
    thinly sliced

½ red onion, thinly
    sliced

1 avocado, sliced

2 radishes, thinly
    sliced

3 tablespoons red
    wine vinegar

  Salt and black
    pepper

3 cups chopped
    lettuce or mixed
    greens

¼ cup crumbled goat
    cheese or feta
    cheese

1 Combine 1 tablespoon oil, 1 teaspoon salt, oregano, paprika, ¼ teaspoon black pepper and 1 clove garlic in large bowl. Rub mixture all over both sides of chicken.

2 Heat 2 tablespoons oil in large skillet over medium-high heat. Add chicken; cook 10 minutes or until no longer pink in center (165°F), turning once.

3 Meanwhile, cook pasta in large saucepan of salted boiling water according to package directions for al dente. Drain and place in large bowl. Add tomatoes, cucumber, onion, avocado and radishes.

4 Whisk remaining ⅓ cup oil, vinegar and remaining 1 clove garlic in small bowl. Season to taste with salt and black pepper. Pour over pasta mixture; stir gently to coat. Stir in lettuce; sprinkle with cheese. Serve with chicken.

MAKES 4 SERVINGS

¼ OF TOTAL RECIPE PER SERVING:

calories 720

total fat 42g

saturated fat 8g

sodium 690mg

carbs 56g

fiber 8g

sugar 5g

protein 38g

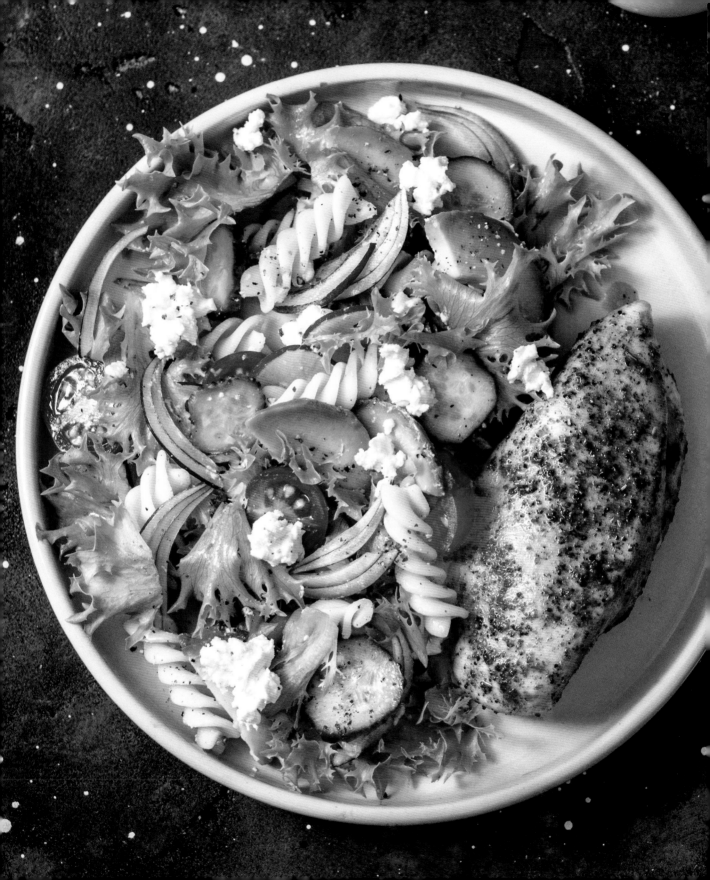

Brown Rice with Chickpeas, Spinach and Feta

½ **cup diced celery**

½ **cup uncooked instant brown rice**

1 **can (about 15 ounces) chickpeas, rinsed and drained**

1 **clove garlic, minced (optional)**

1 **package (10 ounces) frozen chopped spinach, thawed and squeezed dry**

1 **teaspoon Greek or Italian seasoning**

¼ **teaspoon salt (optional)**

⅛ **teaspoon black pepper**

2 **cups water**

½ **cup crumbled reduced-fat feta cheese**

1 **tablespoon lemon juice**

1 Spray large skillet with nonstick cooking spray; heat over medium-high heat. Add celery; cook 4 minutes or until lightly glazed and brown in spots, stirring occasionally.

2 Add rice, chickpeas, garlic, if desired, spinach, Greek seasoning, salt, if desired, and pepper. Stir in water.

3 Cover and bring to a boil. Reduce heat to low; simmer 12 minutes or until rice is tender. Remove from heat; stir in cheese and lemon juice.

MAKES 4 SERVINGS

1 CUP PER SERVING:

calories **190**

total fat **3g**

saturated fat **0g**

sodium **630mg**

carbs **29g**

fiber **7g**

sugar **3g**

protein **16g**

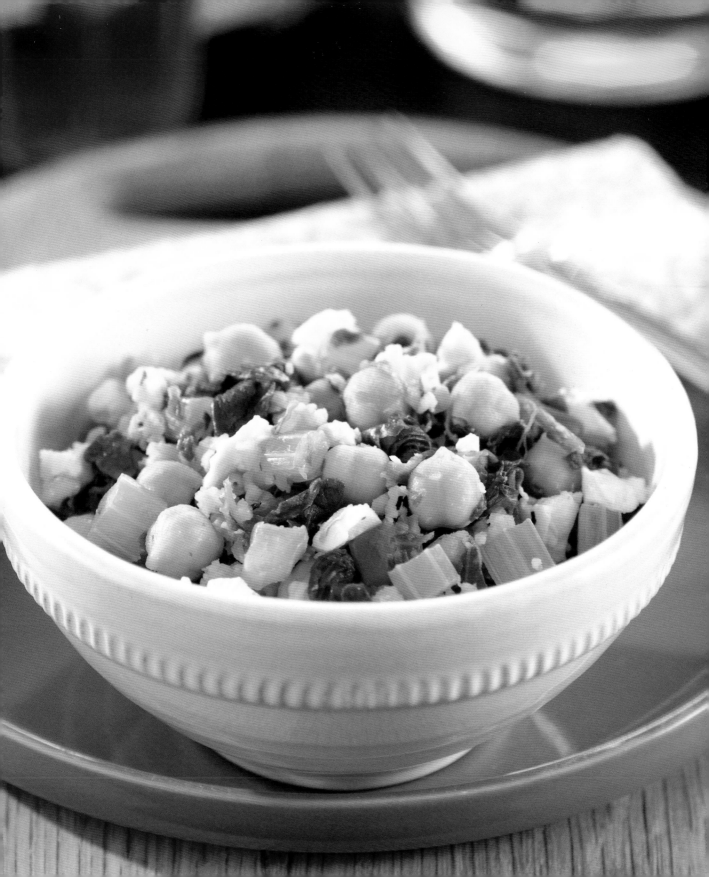

Spicy Chicken Rigatoni

1 **package (16 ounces) uncooked mezzo rigatoni, rigatoni or penne pasta**

¾ **cup frozen peas**

2 **tablespoons olive oil**

2 **cloves garlic, minced**

½ **teaspoon red pepper flakes**

½ **teaspoon black pepper**

8 **ounces boneless skinless chicken breasts, cut into thin strips**

1 **cup marinara sauce**

¾ **cup Alfredo sauce**

Grated Parmesan cheese (optional)

1 Cook pasta in large saucepan of salted boiling water according to package directions for al dente, adding peas during last minute of cooking. Drain and return to saucepan; keep warm.

2 Meanwhile, heat oil in large saucepan over medium-high heat. Add garlic, red pepper flakes and black pepper; cook and stir 1 minute. Add chicken; cook and stir 4 minutes or until cooked through.

3 Add marinara sauce and Alfredo sauce; stir until blended. Reduce heat to medium-low; cook 10 minutes, stirring occasionally.

4 Add pasta and peas; stir gently to coat. Cook 2 minutes or until heated through. Sprinkle with cheese, if desired.

MAKES 6 SERVINGS

$\frac{1}{6}$ **OF TOTAL RECIPE PER SERVING:**

calories **460**

total fat **13g**

saturated fat **4g**

sodium **390mg**

carbs **63g**

fiber **2g**

sugar **6g**

protein **20g**

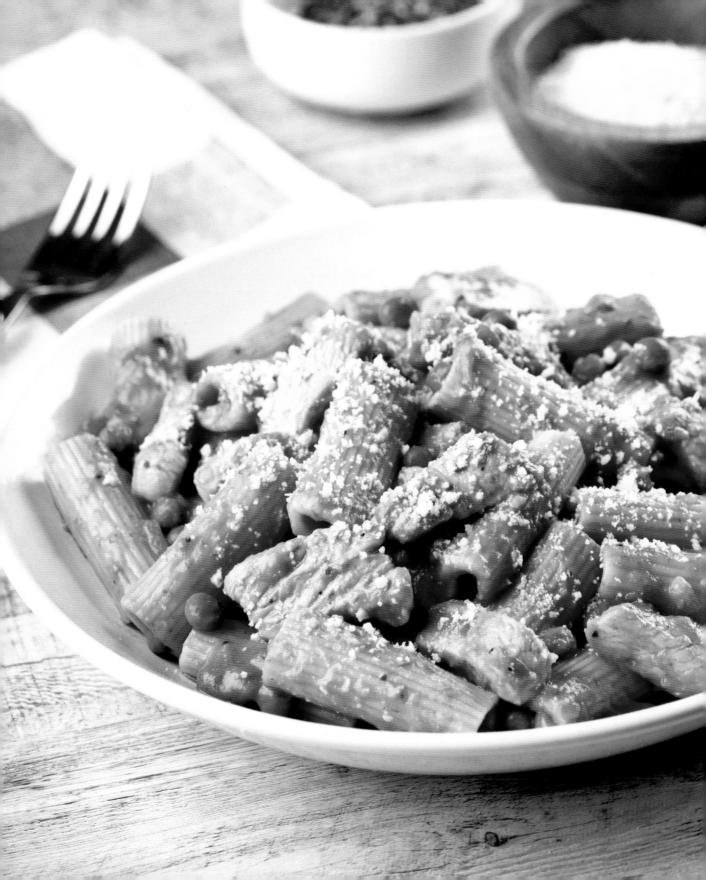

Grilled Fruits with Orange Couscous

2⅔ cups water

1⅓ cups uncooked couscous

½ teaspoon ground cinnamon

½ cup orange juice

2 tablespoons vegetable oil, divided

1 tablespoon soy sauce

1 tablespoon maple syrup

⅛ teaspoon ground nutmeg

½ cup raisins

½ cup chopped walnuts or pecans

Salt and black pepper

2 ripe mangoes, quartered

½ fresh pineapple, cut into ½-inch slices

1 Prepare grill for direct cooking.

2 Bring water to a boil in medium saucepan. Stir in couscous and cinnamon. Remove from heat; cover and let stand 5 minutes. Transfer couscous to large bowl; cool 5 minutes.

3 Meanwhile, blend orange juice, 1 tablespoon oil, soy sauce and maple syrup in glass measuring cup. Blend remaining 1 tablespoon oil and nutmeg in small bowl.

4 Stir orange juice mixture, raisins and walnuts into couscous; season with salt and pepper.

5 Spray grid with nonstick cooking spray. Place mangoes, skin side down, and pineapple on prepared grid. Brush fruits with nutmeg mixture.

6 Grill over medium-high heat 5 to 7 minutes or until fruit is softened, turning pineapple halfway through grilling time. Serve fruit with couscous.

MAKES 4 SERVINGS

¼ OF TOTAL RECIPE PER SERVING:

calories 539

total fat 17g

saturated fat 2g

sodium 268mg

carbs 88g

fiber 7g

sugar 34g

protein 13g

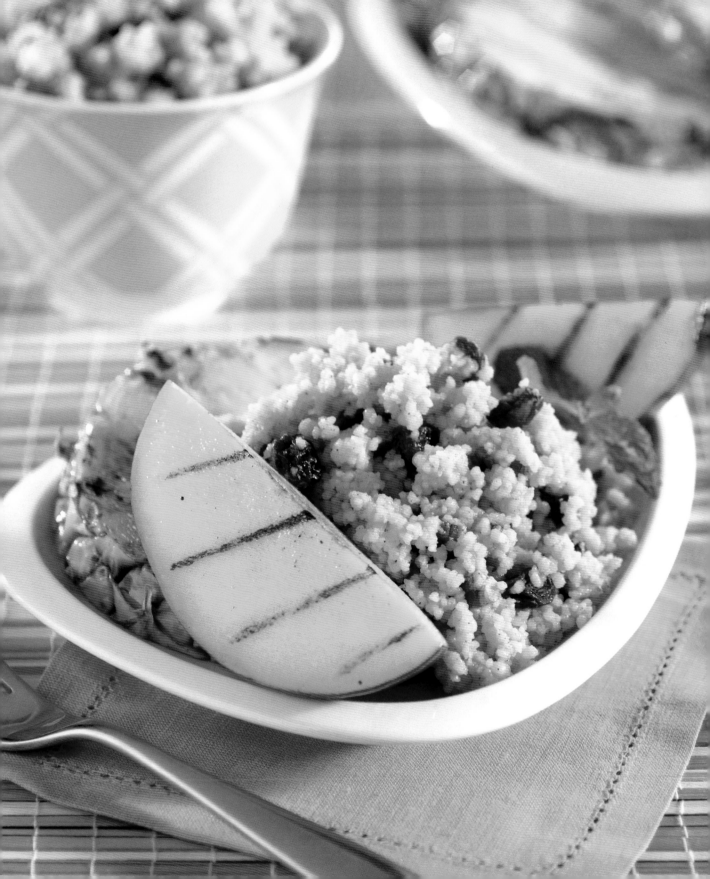

Green Bean, Walnut and Blue Cheese Pasta Salad

2 **cups uncooked gemelli pasta**

2 **cups trimmed halved green beans**

3 **tablespoons olive oil**

2 **tablespoons white wine vinegar**

1 **tablespoon chopped fresh thyme** *or* **1 teaspoon dried thyme**

1 **tablespoon Dijon mustard**

1 **tablespoon lemon juice**

1 **teaspoon honey**

¼ **teaspoon salt**

¼ **teaspoon black pepper**

½ **cup chopped walnuts, toasted***

½ **cup reduced-fat crumbled blue cheese**

*To toast walnuts, cook in medium skillet over medium heat 3 to 4 minutes or until lightly browned and fragrant, stirring frequently.

1 Cook pasta in large saucepan of salted boiling water according to package directions for al dente, adding green beans during last 4 minutes of cooking. Drain and place in large bowl.

2 Meanwhile, whisk oil, vinegar, thyme, mustard, lemon juice, honey, salt and pepper in medium bowl until smooth and well blended.

3 Pour dressing over pasta and green beans; toss to coat evenly. Stir in walnuts and cheese. Serve warm or cover and refrigerate until ready to serve.**

**If serving cold, stir walnuts into salad just before serving.

MAKES 4 SERVINGS

1½ CUPS PER SERVING:

calories 462

total fat 24g

saturated fat 2g

sodium 238mg

carbs 50g

fiber 4g

sugar 3g

protein 14g

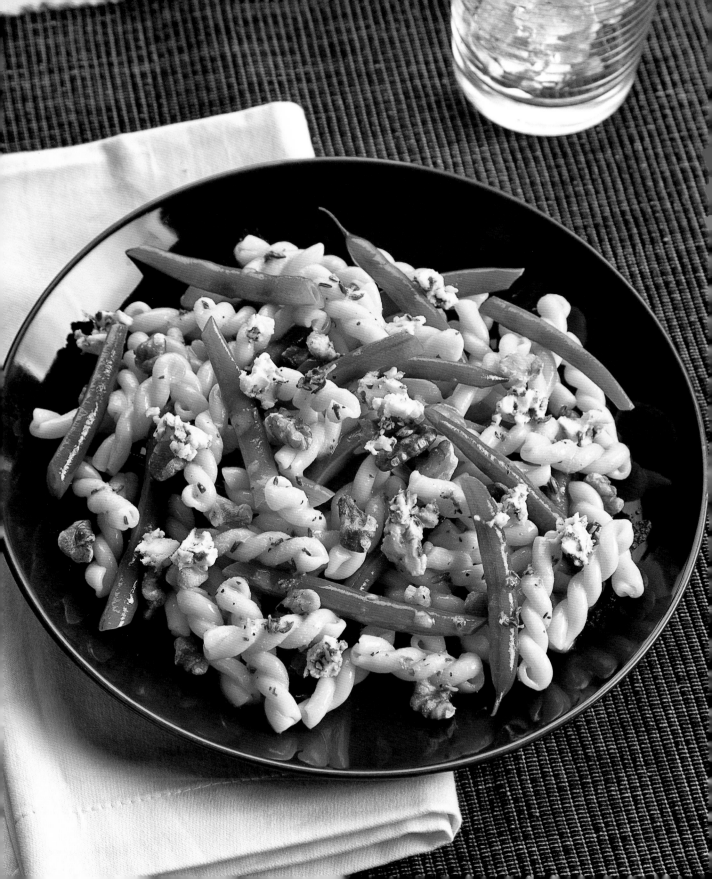

Pasta and White Bean Casserole

MAKES 6 SERVINGS

1/6 OF TOTAL RECIPE PER SERVING:

calories 310

total fat 8g

saturated fat 3g

sodium 870mg

carbs 45g

fiber 7g

sugar 4g

protein 18g

1 tablespoon olive oil

½ cup chopped onion

2 cloves garlic, minced

2 cans (about 15 ounces each) cannellini beans, rinsed and drained

3 cups cooked small shell pasta

1 can (8 ounces) tomato sauce

1½ teaspoons Italian seasoning

½ teaspoon salt

½ teaspoon black pepper

1 cup (4 ounces) shredded Italian cheese blend

2 tablespoons finely chopped fresh parsley

1 Preheat oven to 350°F. Spray 2-quart baking dish with nonstick cooking spray.

2 Heat oil in large skillet over medium-high heat. Add onion and garlic; cook and stir 5 minutes or until onion is softened.

3 Add beans, pasta, tomato sauce, Italian seasoning, salt and pepper; mix well. Transfer to prepared baking dish; sprinkle with cheese and parsley.

4 Bake 20 minutes or until cheese is melted.

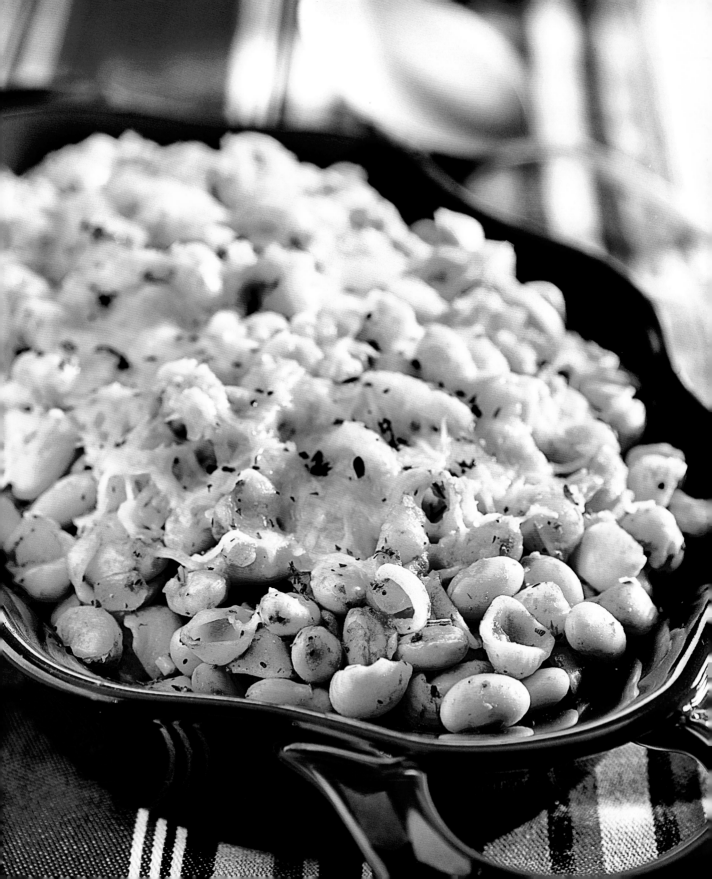

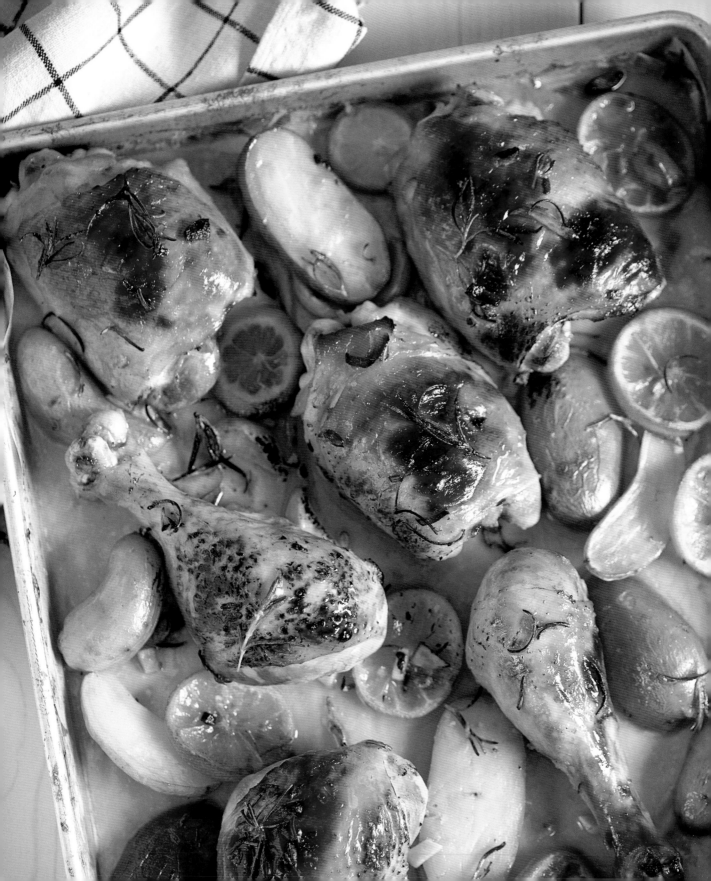

CHICKEN & FISH

Honey Lemon Garlic Chicken

- **2 lemons, divided**
- **2 tablespoons butter, melted**
- **2 tablespoons honey**
- **3 cloves garlic, chopped**
- **2 fresh rosemary sprigs, leaves removed from stems**
- **1 teaspoon coarse salt**
- **½ teaspoon black pepper**
- **3 pounds chicken (4 bone-in skin-on chicken thighs and 4 drumsticks)**
- **1¼ pounds small potatoes, cut into halves or quarters**

1 Preheat oven to 375°F. Grate peel and squeeze juice from 1 lemon. Cut remaining lemon into slices.

2 Combine lemon peel, lemon juice, butter, honey, garlic, rosemary leaves, salt and pepper in small bowl; mix well. Combine chicken, potatoes and lemon slices in large bowl. Pour butter mixture over chicken mixture; toss to coat. Arrange in single layer on large rimmed baking sheet or in shallow roasting pan.

3 Bake about 1 hour or until potatoes are tender and chicken is cooked through (165°F). Cover loosely with foil if chicken skin is browning too quickly.

MAKES 4 SERVINGS

¼ OF TOTAL RECIPE PER SERVING:

calories 440
total fat 15g
saturated fat 6g
sodium 700mg
carbs 36g
fiber 4g
sugar 11g
protein 44g

Lime-Poached Fish with Corn and Chile Salsa

4 **swordfish steaks, 1 inch thick (about 1½ pounds)***

1 **cup baby carrots, cut lengthwise into halves**

2 **green onions, cut into 1-inch pieces**

3 **tablespoons lime juice**

½ **teaspoon salt, divided**

½ **teaspoon chili powder**

1½ **cups chopped tomatoes**

1 **cup frozen corn, thawed**

1 **can (4 ounces) chopped green chiles, drained**

2 **tablespoons chopped fresh cilantro**

1 **tablespoon butter**

*Tuna or halibut steaks can be substituted.

1 Place fish and carrots in saucepan just large enough to hold them in single layer. Add green onions, lime juice, ¼ teaspoon salt and chili powder. Add enough water to just cover fish.

2 Bring to a simmer over medium heat. Cook 8 minutes or until center of fish begins to flake when tested with fork. Transfer fish to serving plates with spatula.

3 Meanwhile for salsa, combine tomatoes, corn, chiles, cilantro and remaining ¼ teaspoon salt in medium bowl; toss well.

4 Drain carrots; add butter. Transfer to serving plates; serve with salsa.

MAKES 4 SERVINGS

¼ OF TOTAL RECIPE PER SERVING:

calories 310

total fat 13g

saturated fat 5g

sodium 590mg

carbs 16g

fiber 3g

sugar 5g

protein 32g

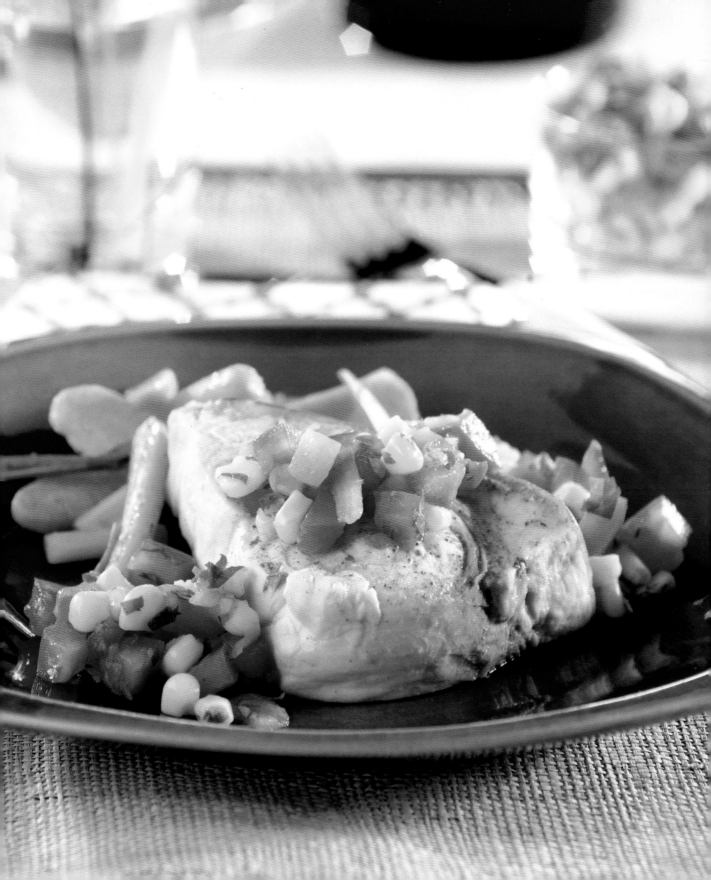

Chicken Tikka Masala Meatballs

MEATBALLS

- **1 pound ground chicken**
- **½ cup plain dry bread crumbs**
- **¼ cup finely chopped onion**
- **1 egg**
- **2 tablespoons chopped fresh cilantro**
- **1 tablespoon minced fresh ginger**
- **1 tablespoon tomato paste**
- **2 cloves garlic, minced**
- **½ teaspoon salt**

TIKKA MASALA SAUCE

- **2 teaspoons sugar**
- **2 teaspoons ground coriander**
- **1 teaspoon ground cumin**
- **½ teaspoon salt**
- **½ teaspoon ground mustard seed**
- **½ teaspoon ground red pepper**
- **1 tablespoon vegetable oil**
- **½ cup finely chopped onion**
- **2 tablespoons minced fresh ginger**
- **3 cloves garlic, minced**
- **1 medium tomato, finely diced**
- **½ cup water**
- **½ cup canned light coconut milk**
- **1 tablespoon tomato paste**
- **¼ cup chopped fresh cilantro**

1 Preheat oven to 400°F. Line large baking sheet with parchment paper.

2 Combine chicken, bread crumbs, ¼ cup onion, egg, 2 tablespoons cilantro, 1 tablespoon ginger, 1 tablespoon tomato paste, 2 cloves garlic and ½ teaspoon salt in large bowl; mix well. Shape into 30 tablespoon-size meatballs. Place on prepared baking sheet. Bake 20 minutes or until cooked through (165°F). Keep warm.

3 Combine sugar, coriander, cumin, salt, mustard and ground red pepper in small bowl.

4 Heat oil in medium saucepan over medium heat. Add ½ cup onion; cook and stir 5 minutes or until just beginning to brown. Add 2 tablespoons ginger, spice mixture and 3 cloves garlic; cook and stir 1 minute. Add tomato, water, coconut milk and 1 tablespoon tomato paste. Reduce heat to low; cook 10 minutes to allow flavors to develop. Add meatballs to saucepan; gently stir to coat evenly.

5 Spoon meatballs onto serving plates; sprinkle with ¼ cup cilantro.

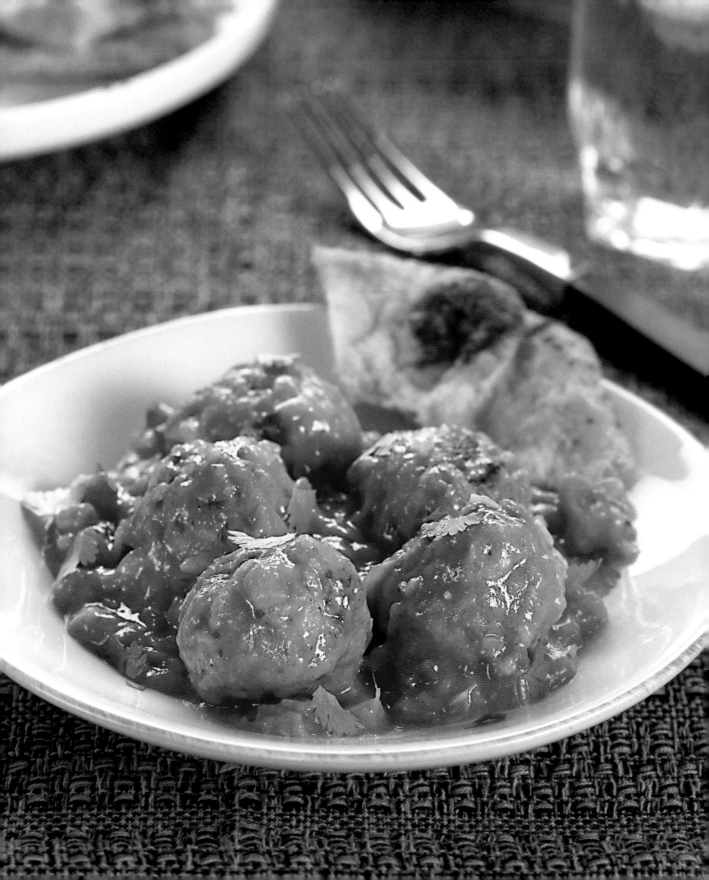

Island Fish Tacos

COLESLAW

- **1 medium jicama (about 12 ounces), peeled and shredded**
- **2 cups packaged coleslaw mix**
- **3 tablespoons finely chopped fresh cilantro**
- **¼ cup lime juice**
- **¼ cup vegetable oil**
- **3 tablespoons white vinegar**
- **2 tablespoons mayonnaise**
- **1 tablespoon honey**
- **½ teaspoon salt**

SALSA

- **2 medium fresh tomatoes, diced (about 2 cups)**
- **½ cup finely chopped red onion**
- **¼ cup finely chopped fresh cilantro**
- **2 tablespoons lime juice**
- **2 tablespoons minced jalapeño pepper**
- **½ teaspoon salt**

TACOS

- **1 to 1¼ pounds white fish such as tilapia or mahi mahi, cut into 3×1½-inch pieces**
- **Salt and black pepper**
- **2 tablespoons vegetable oil**
- **12 (6-inch) tortillas, warmed**
- **Prepared guacamole (optional)**

1 For coleslaw, combine jicama, coleslaw mix and 3 tablespoons cilantro in medium bowl. Whisk ¼ cup lime juice, ¼ cup oil, vinegar, mayonnaise, honey and ½ teaspoon salt in small bowl until well blended. Pour over vegetable mixture; stir to coat. Let stand at least 15 minutes for flavors to blend.

2 For salsa, place tomatoes in fine-mesh strainer; set in bowl or sink to drain 15 minutes. Remove to another medium bowl. Stir in onion, ¼ cup cilantro, 2 tablespoons lime juice, jalapeño and ½ teaspoon salt; mix well.

3 For tacos, season both sides of fish with salt and black pepper. Heat 1 tablespoon oil in large nonstick skillet over medium-high heat. Add half of fish; cook 2 minutes per side or until fish is opaque and begins to flake when tested with fork. Repeat with remaining oil and fish.

4 Break fish into bite-size pieces; serve in tortillas with coleslaw, salsa and guacamole, if desired.

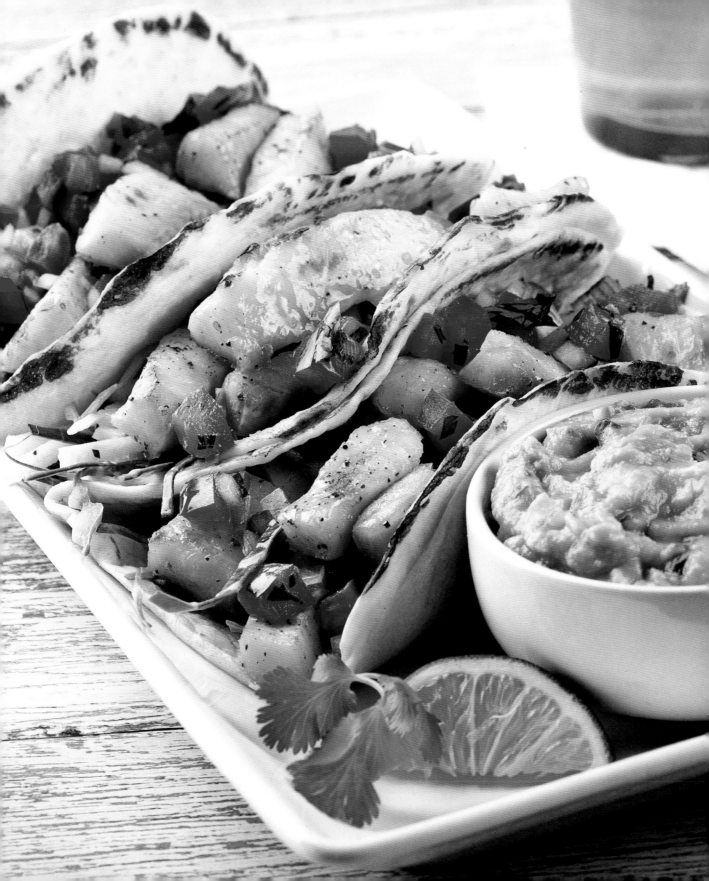

Jambalaya Pasta

- **1 package (16 ounces) uncooked linguine**
- **1 pound boneless skinless chicken breasts, cut into 1-inch pieces**
- **2 tablespoons plus 1 teaspoon Cajun seasoning, divided**
- **1 tablespoon vegetable oil**
- **8 ounces bell peppers (red, yellow, green or a combination), cut into ¼-inch strips**
- **½ medium red onion, cut into ¼-inch strips**
- **6 ounces medium raw shrimp, peeled and deveined**
- **2 cloves garlic, minced**
- **1 teaspoon salt**
- **¼ teaspoon black pepper**
- **1½ pounds plum tomatoes (about 6), cut into ½-inch pieces**
- **1 cup reduced-sodium chicken broth**
- **Chopped fresh parsley**

1 Cook pasta in large saucepan of salted boiling water according to package directions for al dente. Drain and return to saucepan; keep warm.

2 Meanwhile, combine chicken and 2 tablespoons Cajun seasoning in medium bowl; toss to coat. Heat oil in large skillet over medium-high heat. Add chicken; cook and stir 3 minutes.

3 Add bell peppers and onion; cook and stir 3 minutes. Add shrimp, garlic, remaining 1 teaspoon Cajun seasoning, salt and black pepper; cook and stir 1 minute.

4 Stir in tomatoes and broth; bring to a boil. Reduce heat to medium-low; cook 3 minutes or until shrimp are pink and opaque. Serve over hot pasta; sprinkle with parsley.

MAKES 6 SERVINGS

⅙ OF TOTAL RECIPE PER SERVING:

calories 440

total fat 6g

saturated fat 1g

sodium 840mg

carbs 69g

fiber 2g

sugar 6g

protein 28g

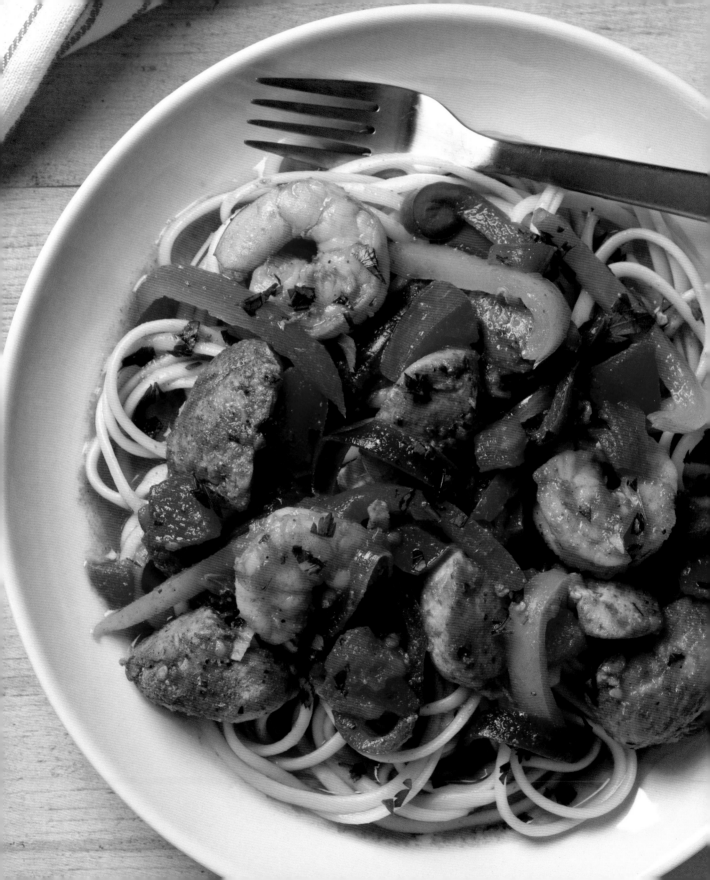

Chicken Marsala

4 boneless skinless
  chicken breasts
  (6 to 8 ounces
  each)
½ cup all-purpose
  flour
1 teaspoon coarse
  salt
¼ teaspoon black
  pepper
2 tablespoons olive
  oil
3 tablespoons butter,
  divided
2 cups (16 ounces)
  sliced mushrooms
1 shallot, minced
1 clove garlic, minced
1 cup dry Marsala
  wine
½ cup chicken broth
  Finely chopped
  fresh parsley

1 Pound chicken to ¼-inch thickness between two sheets of plastic wrap. Combine flour, salt and pepper in shallow dish; mix well. Coat both sides of chicken with flour mixture, shaking off excess.

2 Heat oil and 1 tablespoon butter in large skillet over medium-high heat. Add chicken in single layer; cook 4 minutes per side or until golden brown and cooked through (165°F). Remove to plate; cover loosely with foil to keep warm.

3 Add 1 tablespoon butter, mushrooms and shallot to skillet; cook 10 minutes or until mushrooms are deep golden brown, stirring occasionally. Add garlic; cook and stir 1 minute. Stir in wine and broth; cook 2 minutes, scraping up browned bits from bottom of skillet. Stir in remaining 1 tablespoon butter until melted.

4 Return chicken to skillet; turn to coat with sauce. Cook 2 minutes or until heated through. Sprinkle with parsley.

MAKES 4 SERVINGS

¼ OF TOTAL RECIPE PER SERVING:

calories 520
total fat 20g
saturated fat 7g
sodium 770mg
carbs 25g
fiber 2g
sugar 11g
protein 44g

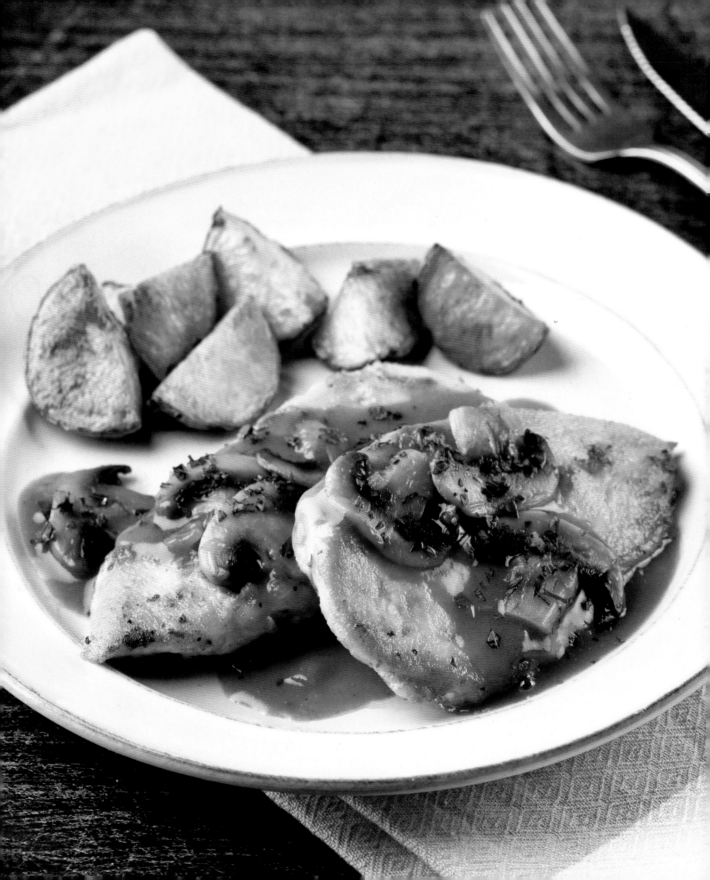

Simple Roasted Chicken

1 **whole chicken (about 4 pounds)**

3 **tablespoons butter, softened**

1½ **teaspoons salt**

1 **teaspoon onion powder**

1 **teaspoon dried thyme**

½ **teaspoon garlic powder**

½ **teaspoon paprika**

½ **teaspoon black pepper**

Fresh parsley sprigs and lemon wedges (optional)

1 Preheat oven to 425°F. Pat chicken dry; place in small baking dish or on baking sheet.

2 Combine butter, salt, onion powder, thyme, garlic powder, paprika and pepper in small microwavable bowl; mash with fork until well blended. Loosen skin on breasts and thighs; spread about one third of butter mixture under skin.

3 Microwave remaining butter mixture until melted. Brush melted butter mixture all over outside of chicken and inside cavity. Tie drumsticks together with kitchen string and tuck wing tips under.

4 Roast 20 minutes. *Reduce oven temperature to 375°F.* Roast 45 to 55 minutes or until chicken is cooked through (165°F), basting once with pan juices during last 10 minutes of cooking time.

5 Transfer chicken to large cutting board; tent with foil. Let stand 15 minutes before carving. Garnish with parsley and lemon wedges.

MAKES 4 SERVINGS

¼ OF TOTAL RECIPE PER SERVING:

calories 360

total fat 20g

saturated fat 8g

sodium 1010mg

carbs 1g

fiber 0g

sugar 0g

protein 43g

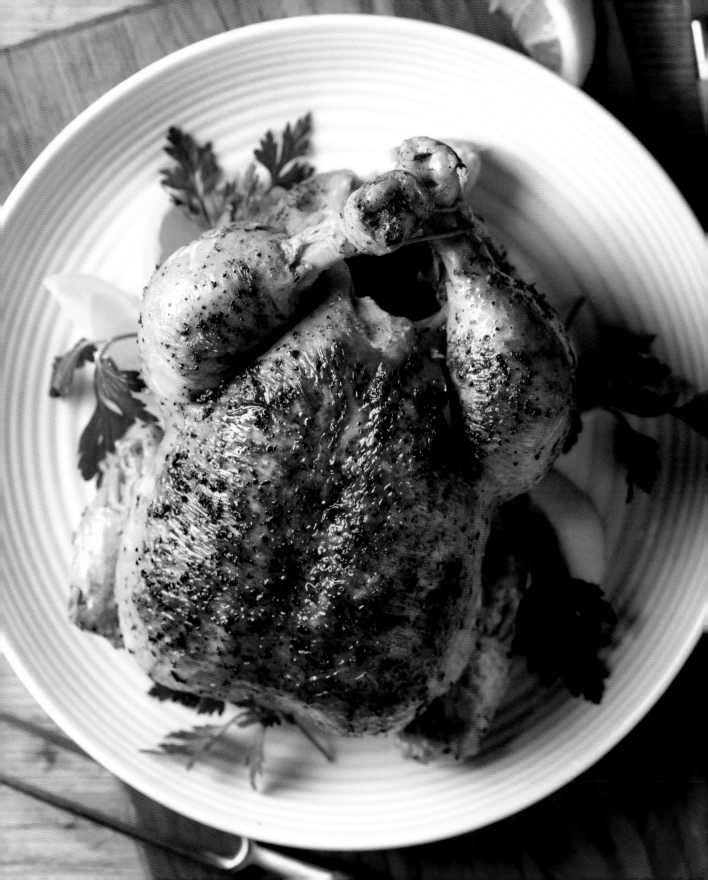

Veggie-Packed Turkey Burgers

1¼ **pounds ground turkey**

½ **cup chopped onion**

½ **cup shredded zucchini**

½ **cup shredded carrots**

1 **teaspoon minced jalapeño pepper**

Salt and black pepper

4 **whole wheat rolls or hamburger buns**

1 **cup shredded lettuce**

8 **tomato slices**

1 Prepare grill for direct cooking over medium-heat. Combine turkey, onion, zucchini, carrots and jalapeño in large bowl. Season with salt and black pepper. Shape into four patties.

2 Grill, covered, 8 to 10 minutes or until cooked through (165°F), turning halfway through grilling.

3 Serve on rolls with lettuce and tomato slices.

MAKES 4 SERVINGS

¼ OF TOTAL RECIPE PER SERVING:

calories 350

total fat 3g

saturated fat 1g

sodium 430mg

carbs 40g

fiber 2g

sugar 5g

protein 41g

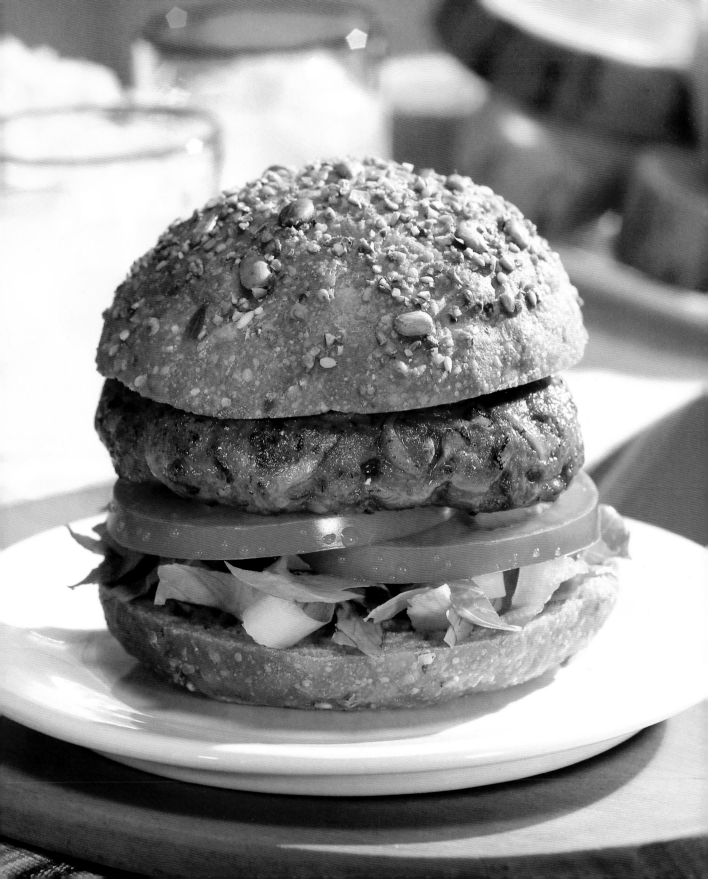

Spatchcock Chicken and Vegetables

1 **whole chicken (about 4 pounds)**

6 **tablespoons (¾ stick) butter, softened**

2 **tablespoons fresh thyme leaves**

1 **tablespoon honey**

1 **tablespoon Dijon mustard**

1¼ **teaspoons salt**

½ **teaspoon black pepper**

12 **ounces small (2-inch) red potatoes, halved (about 12 potatoes)**

8 **ounces parsnips, cut diagonally into 1½-inch pieces (cut in half lengthwise if very thick)**

8 **ounces carrots, cut diagonally into 1½-inch pieces**

1 Position oven rack in lower third of oven. Preheat oven to 425°F. Line baking sheet with foil, if desired.

2 To spatchcock chicken, place breast side down on cutting board. Cut along both sides of backbone with poultry shears or kitchen scissors; remove and discard backbone. Turn chicken breast side up; press down firmly on breast until it cracks to flatten chicken. Place on prepared baking sheet.

3 Combine butter, thyme, honey, mustard, salt and pepper in small microwavable bowl; mix well. Rub 1 tablespoon mixture under skin of chicken breast. Rub 1 tablespoon mixture all over chicken skin.

4 Combine potatoes, parsnips and carrots in large bowl. Melt remaining butter mixture in microwave; pour over vegetables and toss to coat. Arrange vegetables around chicken on baking sheet.

5 Roast 50 to 60 minutes or until chicken is cooked through (165°F), covering chicken loosely with foil after 30 minutes if skin is browning too quickly. Remove chicken to clean cutting board; tent with foil and let stand 10 minutes before slicing. Serve with vegetables.

MAKES 4 SERVINGS

¼ OF TOTAL RECIPE PER SERVING:

calories 580

total fat 29g

saturated fat 14g

sodium 870mg

carbs 34g

fiber 5g

sugar 11g

protein 46g

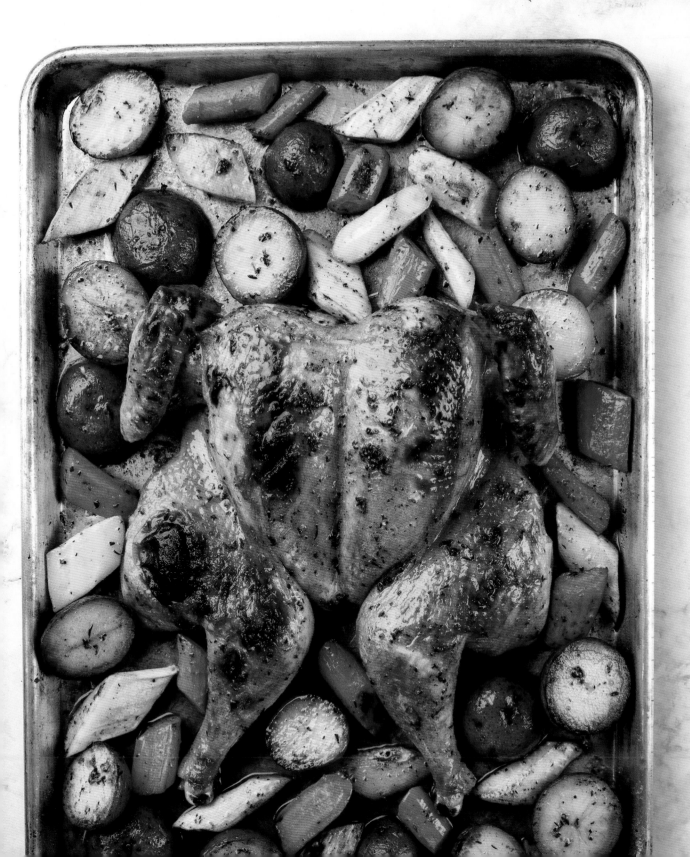

Grilled Salmon Salad

⅓ cup plus
   2 tablespoons fat-free raspberry or balsamic vinaigrette salad dressing, divided

4 **skinless salmon fillets, ¾ inch thick (about 1 pound)**

½ **teaspoon black pepper**

¼ **teaspoon salt**

8 **cups spring mix salad greens**

2 **cups cherry tomatoes, halved**

¼ **cup fresh basil, chopped (optional)**

1 Prepare grill for direct cooking. Brush 2 tablespoons dressing over salmon fillets. Sprinkle with pepper and salt. Grill salmon, covered, over medium-high heat 5 to 6 minutes or until center is opaque.

2 Combine greens, tomatoes and remaining ⅓ cup dressing in large bowl; toss gently. Arrange on four plates. Top with salmon; sprinkle with basil, if desired.

NOTE: To broil the salmon, preheat the broiler. Place salmon on an oiled broiler pan. Broil 4 inches from the heat source 6 to 7 minutes or just until the salmon begins to flake when tested with a fork.

MAKES 4 SERVINGS

1 SALMON FILLET WITH ¼ OF SALAD PER SERVING:

calories 340

total fat 15g

saturated fat 4g

sodium 400mg

carbs 24g

fiber 4g

sugar 17g

protein 25g

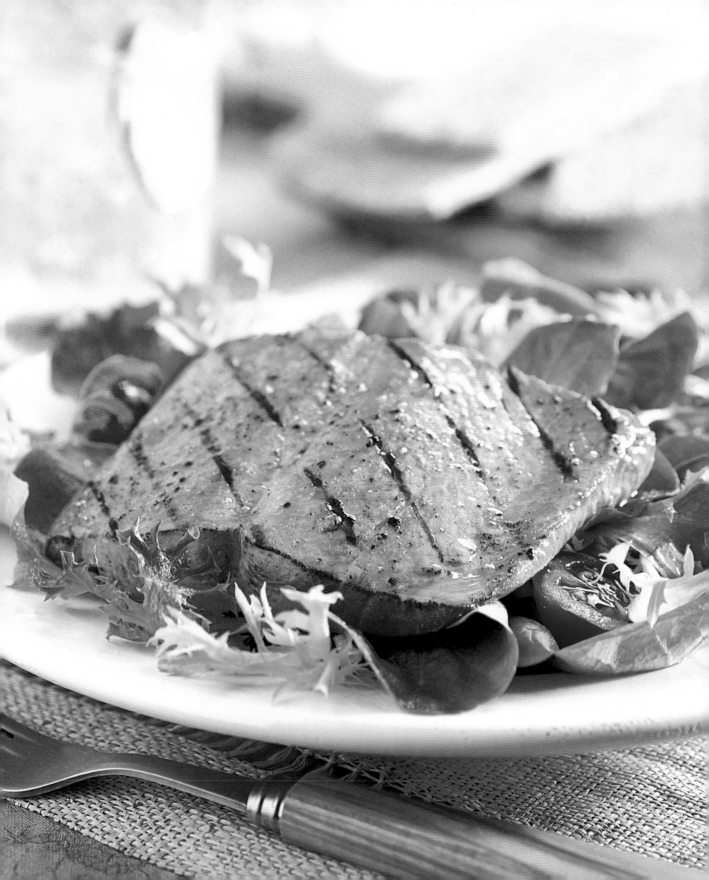

Chicken with Herb Stuffing

- **4 boneless skinless chicken breasts**
- **Salt and black pepper**
- **⅓ cup fresh basil leaves**
- **1 package (8 ounces) goat cheese with garlic and herbs**
- **1 to 2 tablespoons olive oil**

1 Preheat oven to 350°F. Pound chicken to ¼-inch thickness between two sheets of plastic wrap. Season both sides of chicken with salt and pepper.

2 Place basil in food processor; pulse until chopped. Cut goat cheese into large pieces and add to food processor; pulse until combined.

3 Shape about 2 tablespoons of cheese mixture into log and set in center of each chicken breast. Wrap chicken around filling to enclose completely. Tie securely with kitchen string or secure with toothpicks.

4 Heat 1 tablespoon oil in large ovenproof skillet; brown chicken bundles on all sides, adding additional oil as needed to prevent sticking. Place skillet in oven; bake 15 minutes or until chicken is cooked through and filling is hot. Allow to cool slightly, remove string and slice to serve.

MAKES 4 SERVINGS

¼ OF TOTAL RECIPE PER SERVING:

calories 330
total fat 21g
saturated fat 9g
sodium 270mg
carbs 2g
fiber 0g
sugar 2g
protein 36g

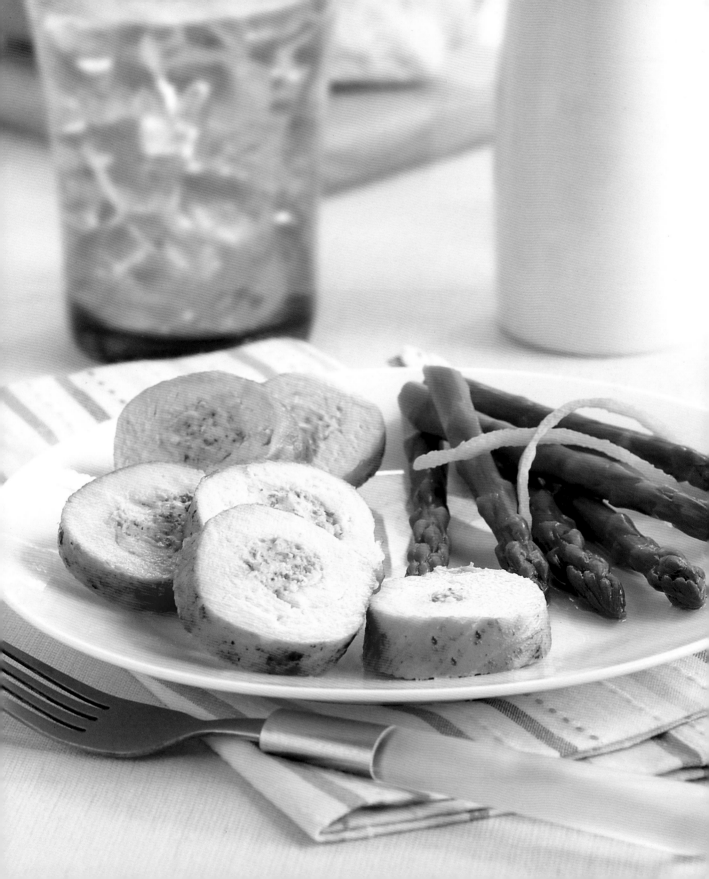

Lemon Butter Chicken

4 **boneless skinless chicken breasts (about 6 ounces each)**

½ **teaspoon salt**

¼ **teaspoon black pepper**

1 **tablespoon olive oil**

6 **tablespoons (¾ stick) butter, divided**

¼ **cup finely chopped onion**

2 **cloves garlic, minced**

½ **cup dry white wine**

¼ **cup lemon juice**

3 **tablespoons thinly sliced oil-packed sun-dried tomatoes (about 4)**

3 **tablespoons slivered fresh basil**

1 **package (4 ounces) goat cheese, cut into 4 pieces**

1 Pound chicken to ½-inch thickness between two sheets of plastic wrap. (Chicken may not need much flattening, but make sure all pieces are even thickness.) Season with salt and pepper.

2 Heat oil in large skillet over medium-high heat. Add chicken; cook 6 to 8 minutes per side or until lightly browned and cooked through (165°F). Remove to plate; tent with foil to keep warm.

3 Add 1 tablespoon butter and onion to skillet; cook and stir 2 minutes or until softened. Add garlic; cook and stir 1 minute. Add wine and lemon juice; bring to a simmer. Cook 10 minutes or until reduced by half.

4 Add remaining 5 tablespoons butter, 1 tablespoon at a time, whisking until smooth. Stir in sun-dried tomatoes and basil; cook just until heated through.

5 Place chicken on serving plates; top with cheese and sauce.

MAKES 4 SERVINGS

¼ OF TOTAL RECIPE PER SERVING:

calories 570
total fat 33g
saturated fat 17g
sodium 770mg
carbs 4g
fiber 1g
sugar 1g
protein 59g

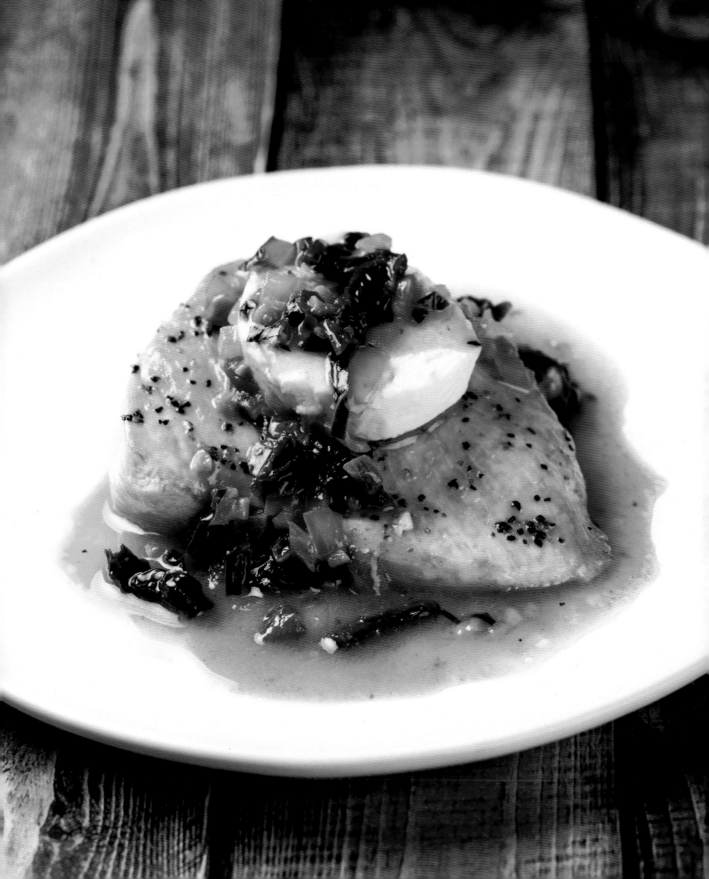

Broiled Cajun Fish Fillets

2 tablespoons all-purpose flour

½ cup seasoned dried bread crumbs

1 teaspoon dried thyme

½ teaspoon garlic salt

¼ teaspoon ground red pepper

¼ teaspoon black pepper

1 egg

1 tablespoon milk or water

4 scrod or orange roughy fillets, ½ inch thick (4 to 5 ounces each)

2 tablespoons butter, melted, divided

⅓ cup mayonnaise

2 tablespoons sweet pickle relish

1 tablespoon lemon juice

1 teaspoon prepared horseradish

1 Preheat broiler. Spray baking sheet with nonstick cooking spray.

2 Place flour in large resealable food storage bag. Combine bread crumbs, thyme, garlic salt, red pepper and black pepper in second bag. Beat egg and milk in shallow dish. Place each fillet, one at a time, in flour; shake bag to coat lightly. Dip fillets into egg mixture, letting excess drip off. Place fillets in bread crumb mixture; shake to coat well. Transfer fillets to prepared baking sheet. Brush fish with 1 tablespoon butter.

3 Broil 4 to 5 inches from heat source 3 minutes. Turn fish; brush with remaining 1 tablespoon butter; broil 3 minutes or until fish begins to flake when tested with fork.

4 Meanwhile, combine mayonnaise, relish, lemon juice and horseradish in small bowl; mix well. Serve sauce with fish.

MAKES 4 SERVINGS

¼ OF TOTAL RECIPE PER SERVING:

calories 370

total fat 22g

saturated fat 6g

sodium 730mg

carbs 17g

fiber 0g

sugar 3g

protein 25g

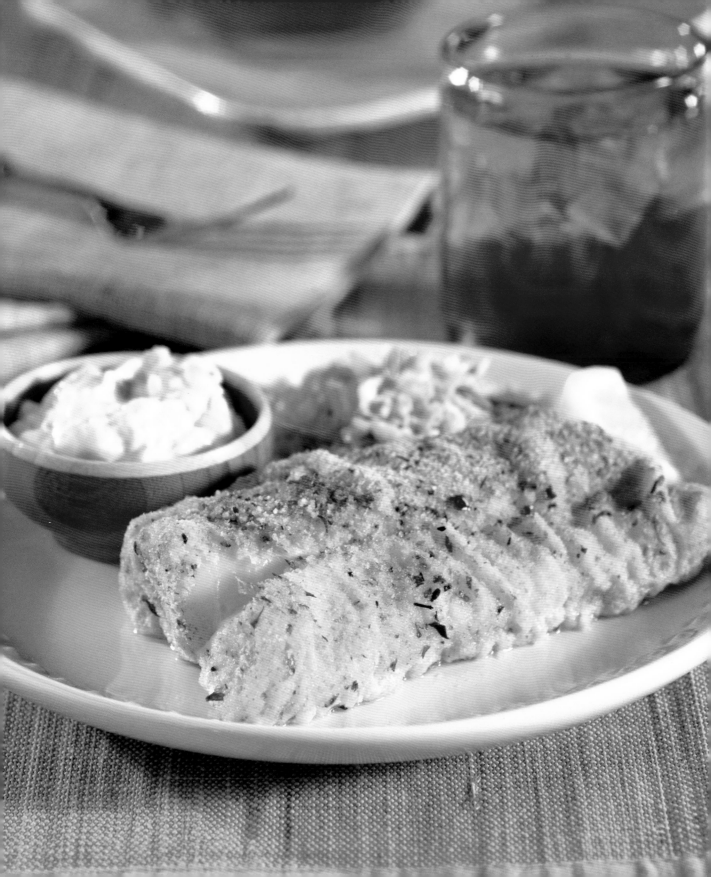

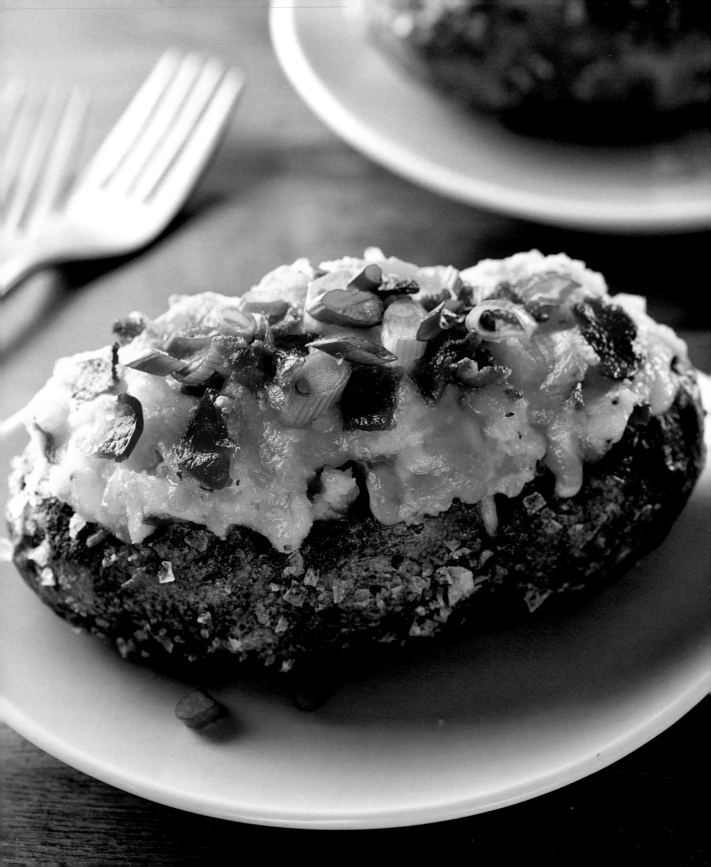

VEGETABLES & SIDES

Loaded Baked Potatoes

- 4 large baking potatoes
- 1 cup (4 ounces) shredded Cheddar cheese*
- 1 cup (4 ounces) shredded Monterey Jack cheese*
- 8 slices bacon, crisp-cooked
- ½ cup sour cream
- ¼ cup (½ stick) butter, melted
- 2 tablespoons milk
- ¼ teaspoon black pepper
  Salt
- 1 tablespoon vegetable oil
- 2 teaspoons coarse salt (optional)
- 1 green onion, thinly sliced (optional)

  Or substitute 2 cups (8 ounces) shredded Cheddar Jack cheese blend for the Cheddar and Monterey Jack cheeses.

1 Preheat oven to 400°F. Prick potatoes all over with fork; place in baking pan. Bake 1 hour or until potatoes are fork-tender. Let stand until cool enough to handle. *Reduce oven temperature to 350°F.*

2 Combine Cheddar and Monterey Jack in small bowl; reserve ¼ cup for garnish. Chop bacon; reserve ¼ cup for garnish.

3 Cut off thin slice from one long side of each potato. Scoop out centers of potatoes, leaving ¼-inch shell. Place flesh from 3 potatoes in medium bowl. (Reserve flesh from fourth potato for another use.) Add sour cream, butter, remaining 1¾ cups shredded cheese, bacon, milk and pepper to bowl with potatoes; mash until well blended. Season to taste with salt.

4 Turn potato shells over; brush bottoms and sides with oil. Sprinkle evenly with coarse salt, if desired. Turn right side up and return to baking pan. Fill shells with mashed potato mixture, mounding over tops of shells. Sprinkle with reserved cheese and bacon.

5 Bake 20 minutes or until filling is hot and cheese is melted. Garnish with green onion.

MAKES 4 SERVINGS

¼ OF TOTAL RECIPE PER SERVING:

calories 640
total fat 43g
saturated fat 24g
sodium 720mg
carbs 41g
fiber 3g
sugar 3g
protein 25g

Balsamic Butternut Squash

3 tablespoons olive oil

2 tablespoons thinly sliced fresh sage (about 6 large leaves), divided

1 medium butternut squash, peeled and cut into 1-inch pieces (4 to 5 cups)

½ red onion, cut into ¼-inch slices

1 teaspoon salt, divided

2½ tablespoons balsamic vinegar

¼ teaspoon black pepper

1 Heat oil in large (12-inch) cast iron skillet over medium-high heat. Add 1 tablespoon sage; cook and stir 3 minutes. Add squash, onion and ½ teaspoon salt; cook 6 minutes, stirring occasionally. Reduce heat to medium; cook 15 minutes without stirring.

2 Stir in vinegar, remaining ½ teaspoon salt and pepper; cook 10 minutes or until squash is tender, stirring occasionally. Stir in remaining 1 tablespoon sage; cook 1 minute.

TIP: Leftover squash is a versatile ingredient to have on hand. Toss leftover cubes in a salad, add it to macaroni and cheese or stir it into chili or soup. Or mash it with a fork and use is as a spread on sandwiches or quesadillas.

MAKES 4 SERVINGS

¼ OF TOTAL RECIPE PER SERVING:

calories 170

total fat 11g

saturated fat 2g

sodium 600mg

carbs 20g

fiber 3g

sugar 6g

protein 2g

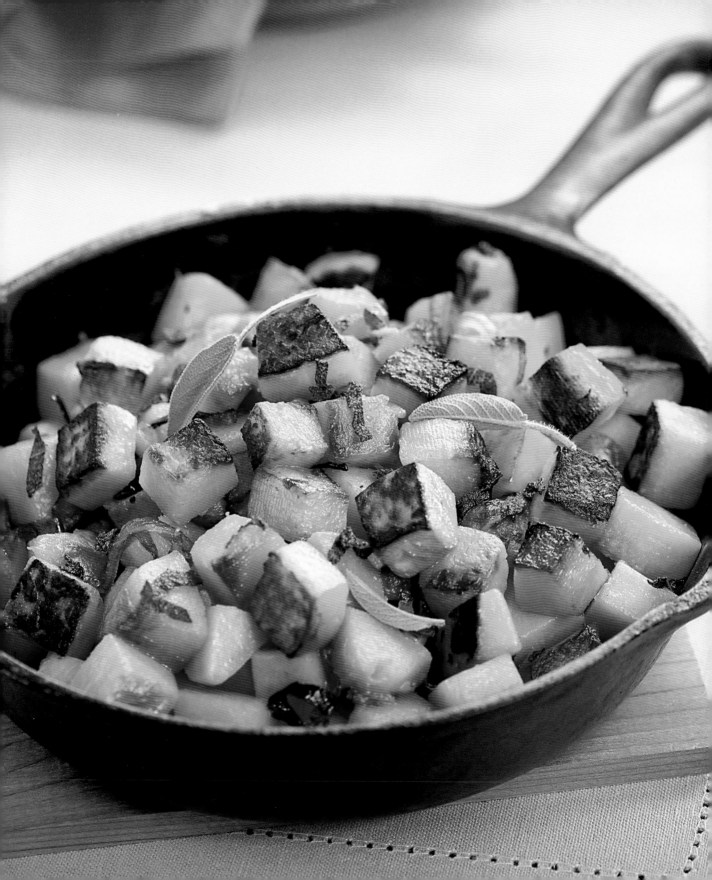

Crunchy Asparagus

1 **bunch fresh asparagus, ends trimmed**

1 **teaspoon lemon juice**

3 **to 4 drops hot pepper sauce**

¼ **teaspoon salt**

¼ **teaspoon dried basil**

Black pepper

2 **teaspoons sunflower kernels**

Lemon slices (optional)

1 Bring about 1 inch of salted water to a simmer in large skillet. Add asparagus; cook 4 minutes or until crisp-tender. Drain and rinse under cold water to stop cooking. Place in serving dish.

2 Combine lemon juice, hot pepper sauce, salt and basil in small bowl. Pour mixture over asparagus; toss to coat. Season with pepper; sprinkle with sunflower kernels. Serve with lemon slices, if desired.

MAKES 4 SERVINGS

¼ OF TOTAL RECIPE PER SERVING:

calories 30
total fat 1g
saturated fat 0g
sodium 170mg
carbs 4g
fiber 1g
sugar 2g
protein 3g

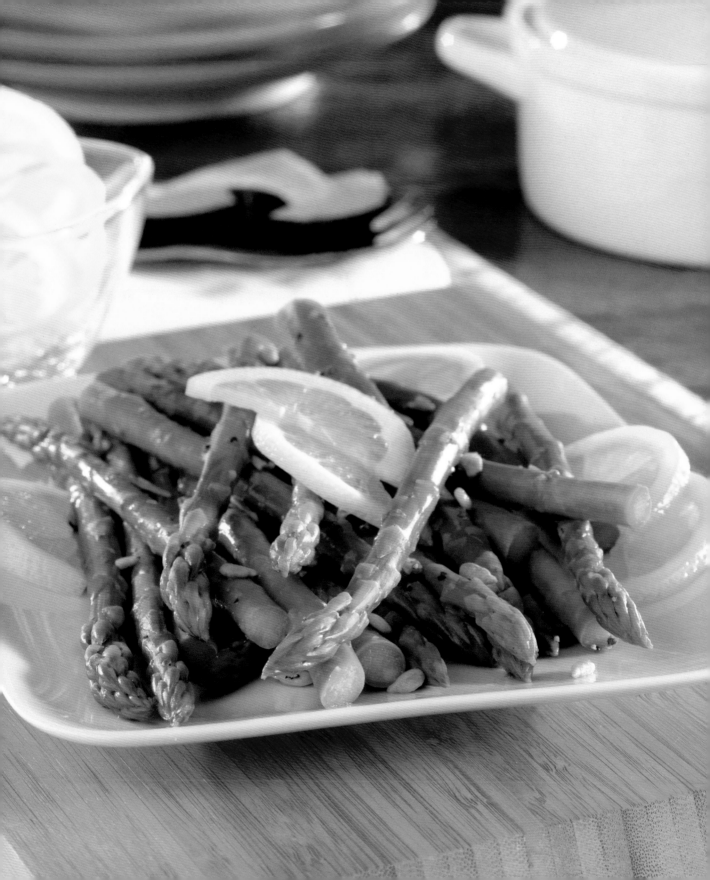

Butternut Squash in Coconut Milk

⅓ cup flaked coconut

2 teaspoons vegetable oil

½ small onion, finely chopped

2 cloves garlic, minced

1 cup unsweetened coconut milk

¼ cup packed brown sugar

1 tablespoon fish sauce or soy sauce

¼ teaspoon salt

⅛ to ¼ teaspoon red pepper flakes

1 butternut squash (2 to 2½ pounds), peeled and cut into large cubes

1 tablespoon chopped fresh cilantro

1 Preheat oven to 350°F. Spread coconut in small baking pan. Bake 6 minutes or until golden, stirring occasionally. Set aside to cool and crisp.

2 Heat oil in large saucepan over medium-high heat. Add onion and garlic; cook and stir 3 minutes or until tender. Add coconut milk, brown sugar, fish sauce, salt and red pepper flakes; stir until brown sugar is dissolved. Bring to a boil; stir in squash.

3 Reduce heat to medium; cover and simmer 30 minutes or until squash is tender. Transfer squash to serving bowl with slotted spoon.

4 Increase heat to high; boil remaining liquid until thick, stirring constantly. Pour liquid over squash in bowl; stir gently to blend. Sprinkle with toasted coconut and cilantro.

MAKES 4 SERVINGS

¼ OF TOTAL RECIPE PER SERVING:

calories 230

total fat 7g

saturated fat 5g

sodium 500mg

carbs 44g

fiber 5g

sugar 21g

protein 4g

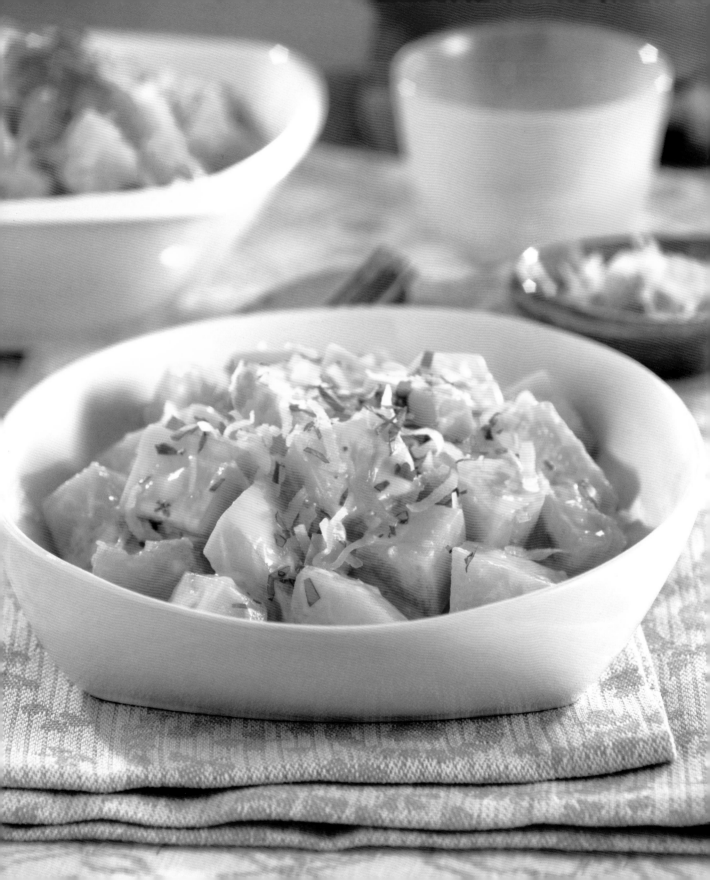

Pumpkin and Parmesan Twice-Baked Potatoes

- **2 baking potatoes (12 ounces each)**
- **1 cup shredded Parmesan cheese, divided**
- **6 tablespoons half-and-half**
- **¼ cup canned pumpkin**
- **1½ teaspoons minced fresh sage *or* ¼ teaspoon dried sage or thyme**
- **¼ teaspoon salt**
- **⅛ teaspoon black pepper**

1 Preheat oven to 400°F. Scrub potatoes; pierce in several places with fork or small knife. Place potatoes directly on oven rack; bake 1 hour or until soft.

2 When cool enough to handle, cut potatoes in half lengthwise. Scoop out centers of potatoes, leaving ¼-inch shell. Place potato flesh in medium bowl; mash with fork. Add ¾ cup cheese, half-and-half, pumpkin, sage, salt and pepper; mix well.

3 Place potato shells on baking sheet; spoon pumpkin mixture into shells. Sprinkle 1 tablespoon of remaining cheese over each potato half. Bake 10 minutes or until filling is heated through.

MAKES 4 SERVINGS

1 FILLED POTATO HALF PER SERVING:

calories 260
total fat 7g
saturated fat 5g
sodium 520mg
carbs 39g
fiber 4g
sugar 4g
protein 13g

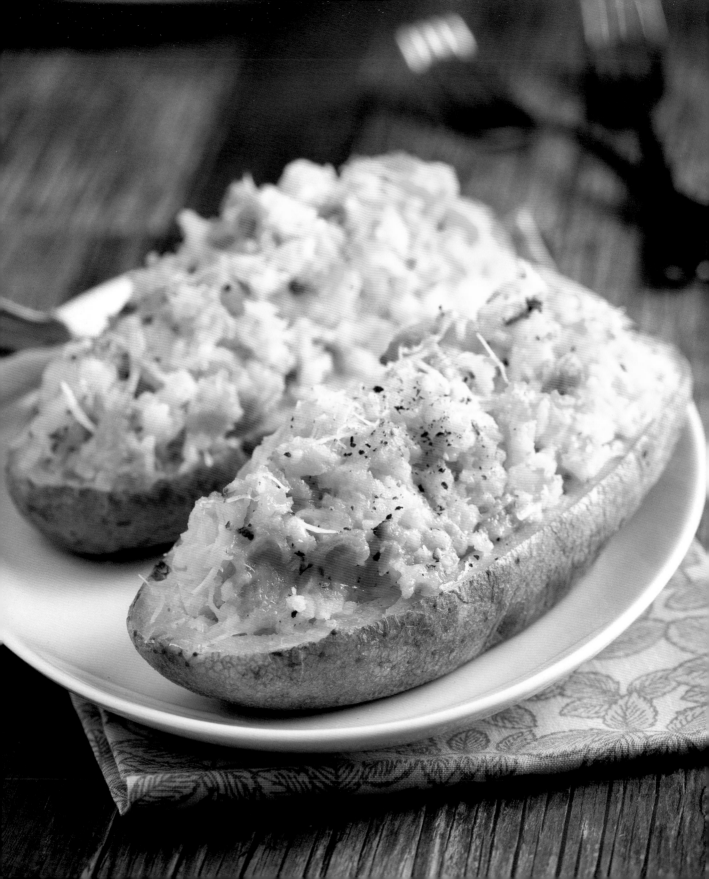

Cauliflower Picnic Salad

1 teaspoon salt

1 head cauliflower,
cut into 1-inch
florets

¾ cup mayonnaise

1 tablespoon yellow
mustard

2 tablespoons minced
fresh parsley

⅓ cup chopped dill
pickle

⅓ cup minced red
onion

2 hard-cooked eggs,
chopped (see Tip)

Salt and black
pepper (optional)

1 Fill large saucepan with 1 inch of water.
Bring to a simmer over medium-high
heat; stir in salt. Add cauliflower; reduce
heat to medium. Cover and cook 5 to
7 minutes or until cauliflower is fork-
tender but not mushy. Drain and cool
slightly.

2 Whisk mayonnaise, mustard and parsley
in large bowl. Stir in pickle and onion.
Gently fold in cauliflower and eggs.
Season with salt and pepper, if desired.

TIP: For hard-cooked eggs, bring
medium saucepan of water to a boil.
Gently add eggs with slotted spoon.
Reduce heat to maintain a simmer;
cook 12 minutes. Meanwhile, fill medium
bowl with cold water and ice cubes.
Drain eggs and place in ice water; cool
10 minutes. Peel when eggs are cool
enough to handle.

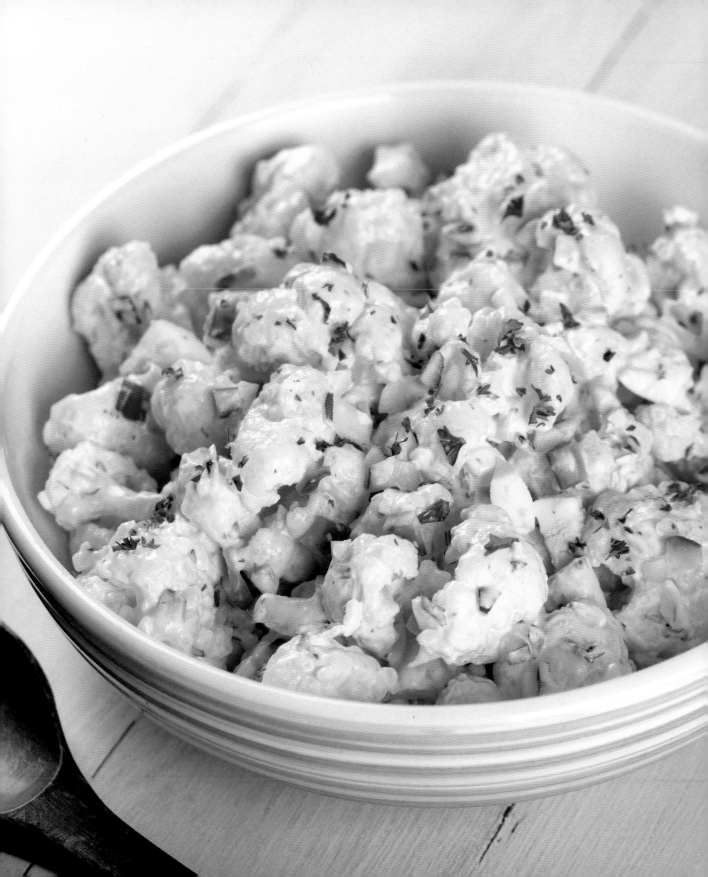

Honey Butter Green Beans

- **1 pound green beans, trimmed**
- **1 pound yellow wax beans, trimmed**
- **2 tablespoons butter**
- **2 tablespoons honey**
- **1 tablespoon grated lemon peel**
- **1 teaspoon salt**
- **½ teaspoon black pepper**
- **1 tablespoon chopped fresh thyme**

1 Bring 10 cups of salted water to a boil in large saucepan. Add beans; boil 2 minutes. Drain and immediately transfer to bowl of ice water or rinse under cold water to stop cooking. Drain and pat dry.*

2 Melt butter in large nonstick skillet over medium-high heat. Add beans; cook and stir 2 minutes or until heated through. Add honey; cook 1 minute. Remove from heat; stir in lemon peel, salt, pepper and thyme. Serve immediately.

This can be done several hours ahead. Cover and refrigerate beans until ready to use.

MAKES 8 SERVINGS

⅛ OF TOTAL RECIPE PER SERVING:

calories 70

total fat 3g

saturated fat 2g

sodium 490mg

carbs 10g

fiber 3g

sugar 7g

protein 2g

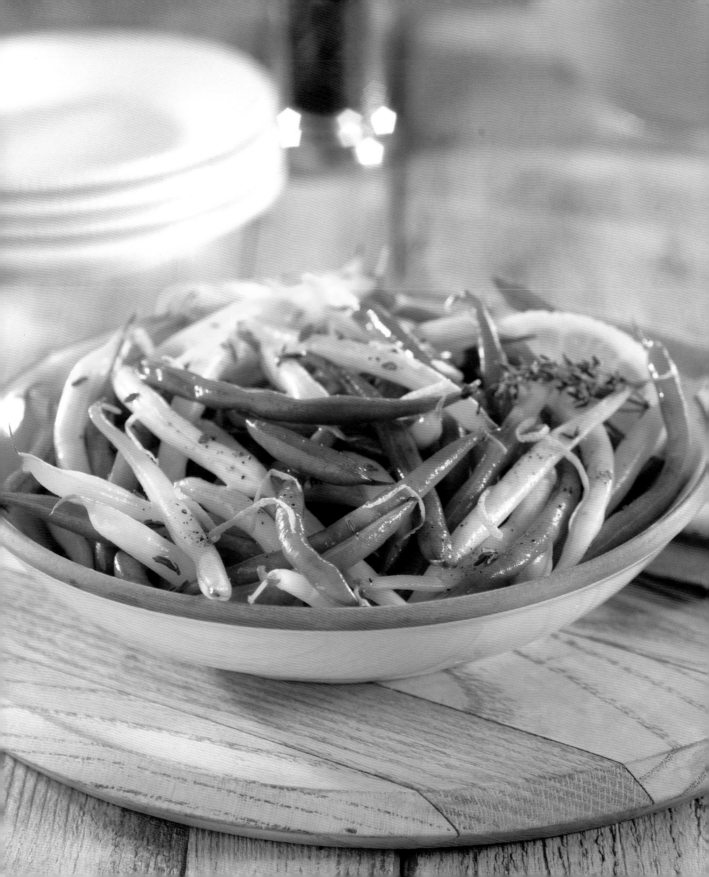

Crispy Smashed Potatoes

1 tablespoon plus ½ teaspoon salt, divided

3 pounds small red potatoes (2 inches or smaller)

4 tablespoons (½ stick) butter, melted, divided

¼ teaspoon black pepper

½ cup grated Parmesan cheese (optional)

1 Fill large saucepan three-fourths full with water; add 1 tablespoon salt. Bring to a boil over high heat. Add potatoes; boil 20 minutes or until potatoes are tender when pierced with tip of sharp knife. Drain potatoes; set aside until cool enough to handle.

2 Preheat oven to 450°F. Brush large baking sheet with 2 tablespoons butter. Working with one potato at a time, smash with hand or bottom of measuring cup to about ½-inch thickness. Arrange smashed potatoes in single layer on prepared baking sheet. Brush with remaining 2 tablespoons butter; sprinkle with remaining ½ teaspoon salt and pepper.

3 Bake 30 to 40 minutes or until bottoms of potatoes are golden brown. Turn potatoes; bake 10 minutes. Sprinkle with cheese, if desired; bake 5 minutes or until cheese is melted.

MAKES ABOUT 6 SERVINGS

⅙ OF TOTAL RECIPE PER SERVING:

calories 230

total fat 8g

saturated fat 5g

sodium 690mg

carbs 36g

fiber 4g

sugar 3g

protein 4g

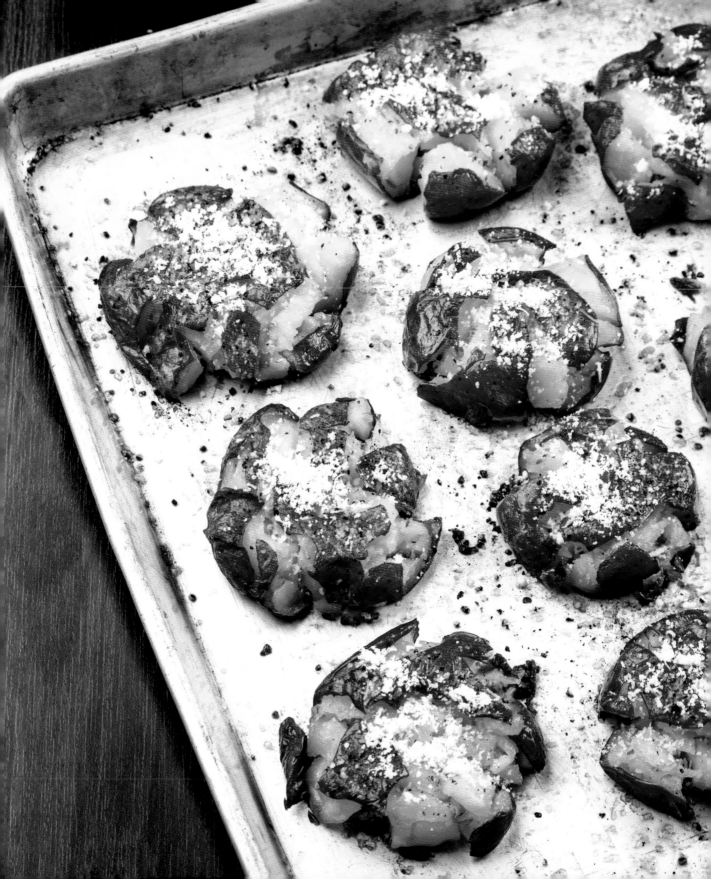

Zucchini with Toasted Chickpea Flour

½ **cup sifted chickpea flour**

1½ **pounds zucchini and/or yellow squash (3 or 4)**

2 **tablespoons olive oil**

1 **tablespoon butter**

1 **tablespoon minced garlic**

1 **teaspoon salt**

½ **teaspoon black pepper**

½ **cup water**

1 Heat large skillet over medium-high heat; add chickpea flour. Cook and stir 3 to 4 minutes or until fragrant and slightly darker in color. Transfer to bowl; wipe out skillet with paper towels.

2 Cut zucchini into ½-inch-thick circles or half moons. Heat oil and butter in same skillet. Add garlic; cook and stir 1 minute or until fragrant. Add zucchini, salt and pepper; cook and stir 5 minutes or until beginning to soften.

3 Stir chickpea flour into skillet to coat zucchini. Pour in water; cook and stir 2 to 3 minutes or until moist crumbs form, scraping bottom of skillet frequently to prevent sticking and scrape up brown bits.

NOTE: Using chickpea flour to add substance and nutrition to vegetable dishes is a method adapted from Indian cuisine. The flour forms delicious, nutty crumbs that become part of the dish. The same method can be used with other vegetables as well.

MAKES 4 SERVINGS

¼ OF TOTAL RECIPE PER SERVING:

calories 170

total fat 12g

saturated fat 3g

sodium 630mg

carbs 12g

fiber 3g

sugar 5g

protein 5g

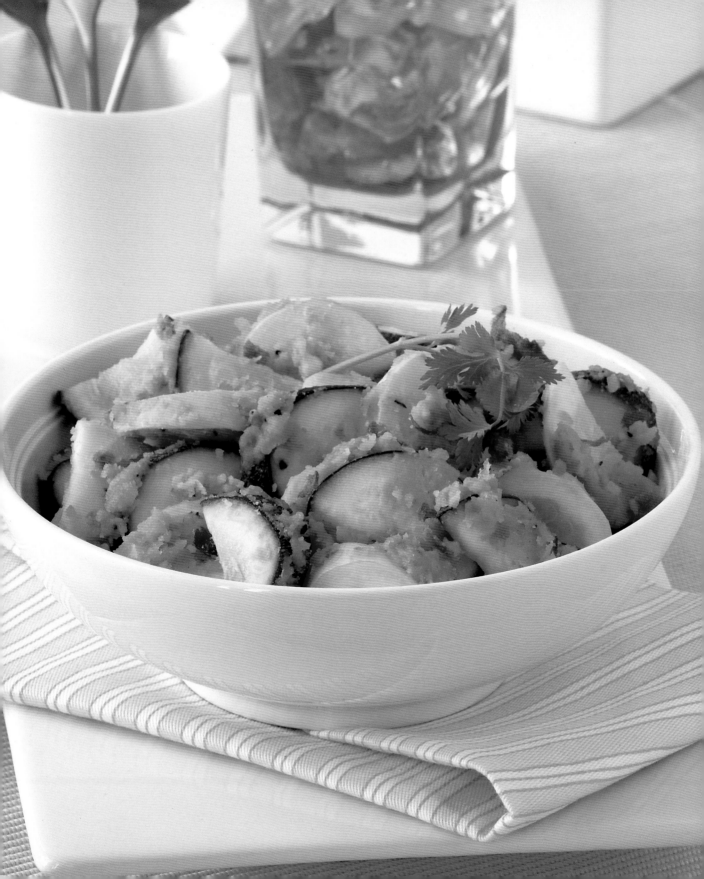

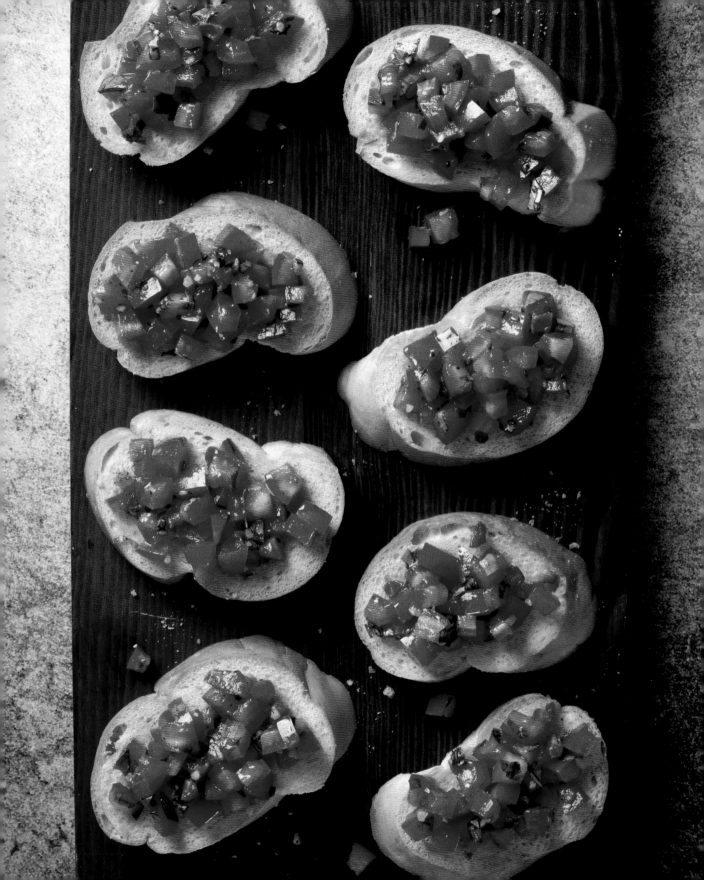

SNACKS & TREATS

Bruschetta

- 4 **plum tomatoes, seeded and diced**
- ½ **cup packed fresh basil leaves, finely chopped**
- 5 **tablespoons olive oil, divided**
- 2 **cloves garlic, minced**
- 2 **teaspoons finely chopped oil-packed sun-dried tomatoes**
- ¼ **teaspoon salt**
- ⅛ **teaspoon black pepper**
- 16 **slices Italian bread**
- 2 **tablespoons grated Parmesan cheese**

1 Combine fresh tomatoes, basil, 3 tablespoons oil, garlic, sun-dried tomatoes, salt and pepper in large bowl; mix well. Let stand at room temperature 1 hour to blend flavors.

2 Preheat oven to 375°F. Place bread on baking sheet. Brush remaining 2 tablespoons oil over one side of bread slices; sprinkle with cheese. Bake 6 to 8 minutes or until toasted.

3 Top each bread slice with 1 tablespoon tomato mixture.

MAKES 8 SERVINGS

2 CROSTINI PER SERVING:

calories 270
total fat 12g
saturated fat 2g
sodium 470mg
carbs 34g
fiber 0g
sugar 7g
protein 5g

Garlic-Parmesan Popcorn

1 tablespoon olive oil

1 clove garlic, finely minced

1 tablespoon light butter-and-oil spread or regular butter, melted

12 cups plain popped popcorn

⅓ cup finely grated Parmesan cheese

½ teaspoon dried basil

½ teaspoon dried oregano

Stir oil and garlic into spread in small bowl until well blended. Pour over popcorn in large bowl; toss to coat. Sprinkle with cheese, basil and oregano.

TIP: One regular-size microwavable package of popcorn yields about 10 to 12 cups of popped popcorn.

MAKES 12 CUPS POPCORN (ABOUT 6 SERVINGS)

2 CUPS PER SERVING:

calories 110

total fat 5g

saturated fat 1g

sodium 83mg

carbs 13g

fiber 2g

sugar 0g

protein 4g

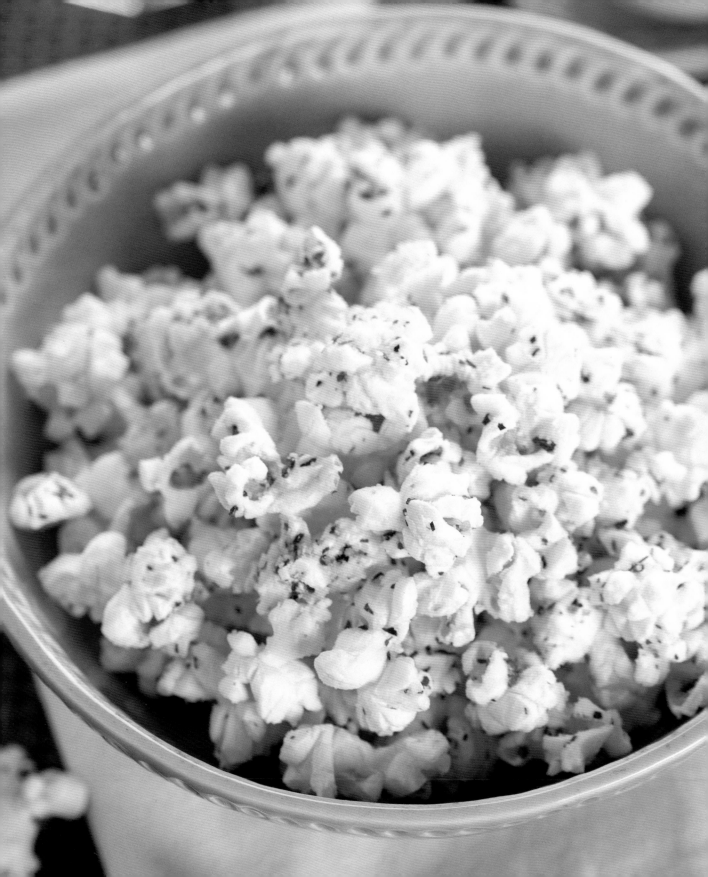

Easy No-Bake Cocoa Oatmeal Cookies

1 cup sugar

1 cup flaked coconut

½ cup unsweetened cocoa powder

½ cup creamy peanut butter

½ cup milk

½ teaspoon vanilla

2 cups old-fashioned oats

1 Line cookie sheet with parchment paper.

2 Combine sugar, coconut, cocoa, peanut butter, milk and vanilla in medium saucepan; bring to a boil over medium-high heat. Reduce heat to low; stir in oats until well blended.

3 Drop dough by tablespoonfuls onto prepared cookie sheet. Freeze 1 to 2 hours or until firm. Store in refrigerator.

MAKES 2 DOZEN COOKIES

2 COOKIES PER SERVING:

calories 220

total fat 9g

saturated fat 4g

sodium 70mg

carbs 34g

fiber 4g

sugar 21g

protein 5g

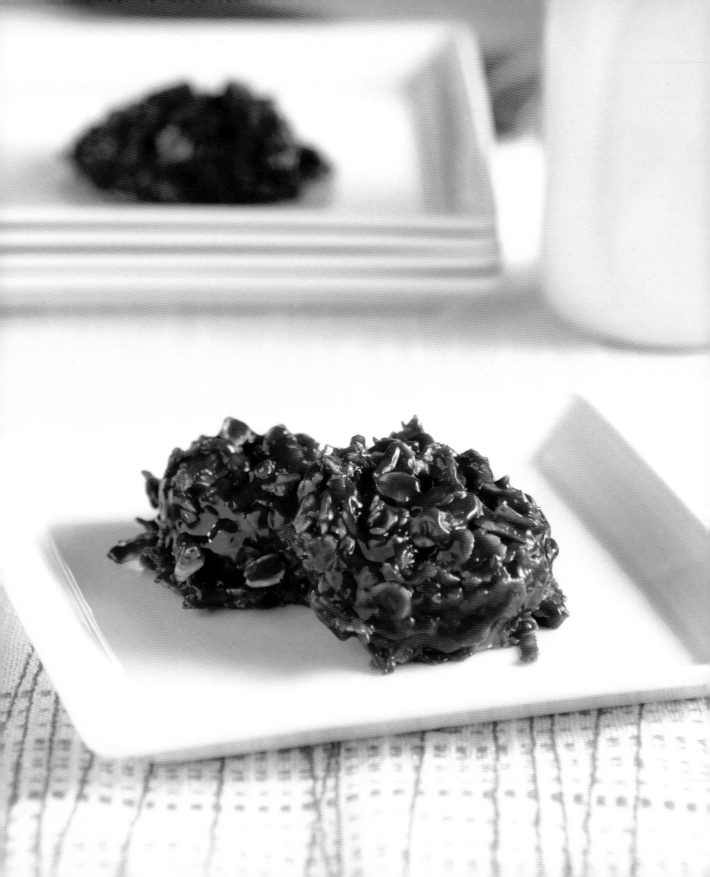

Fruit Kabobs with Raspberry Yogurt Dip

½ cup plain nonfat yogurt

¼ cup raspberry fruit spread

1 pint fresh strawberries

2 cups cubed honeydew melon (1-inch cubes)

2 cups cubed cantaloupe (1-inch cubes)

1 can (8 ounces) pineapple chunks in juice, drained

1 Stir yogurt and fruit spread in small bowl until well blended.

2 Thread fruit alternately onto six 12-inch skewers. Serve with yogurt dip.

MAKES 6 SERVINGS

1 KABOB WITH 2 TABLESPOONS DIP PER SERVING:

calories 110

total fat 0g

saturated fat 0g

sodium 30mg

carbs 27g

fiber 2g

sugar 22g

protein 2g

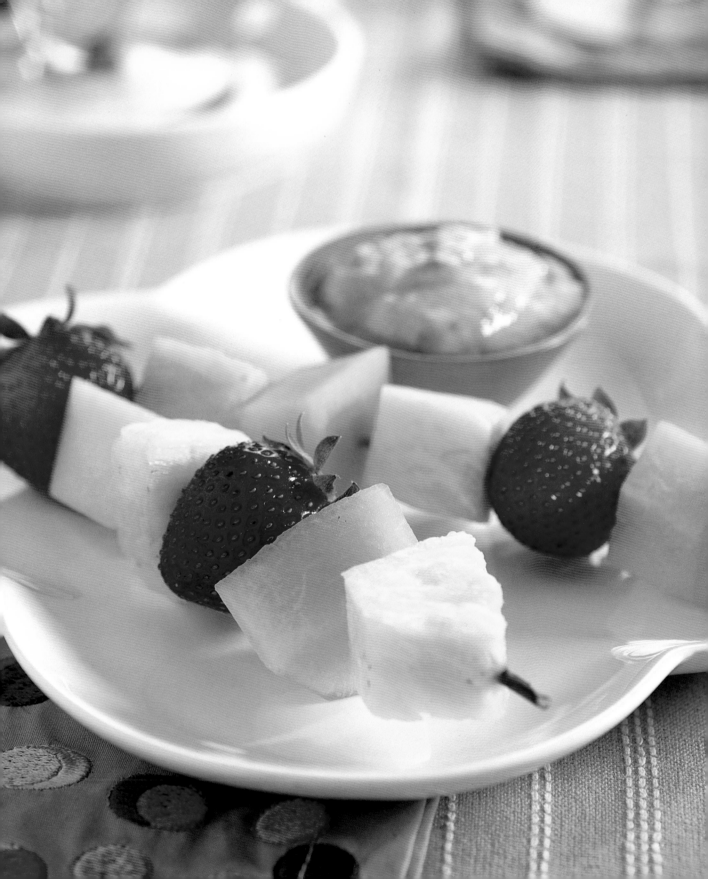

Trail Mix Truffles

⅓ cup dried apples

¼ cup dried apricots

¼ cup apple butter

2 tablespoons golden raisins

1 tablespoon reduced-fat or regular peanut butter

½ cup reduced-fat granola

4 tablespoons graham cracker crumbs, divided

¼ cup mini chocolate chips

1 tablespoon water

1 Combine apples, apricots, apple butter, raisins and peanut butter in food processor or blender; process until smooth. Stir in granola, 1 tablespoon graham cracker crumbs, chocolate chips and water. Shape mixture into 16 balls.

2 Place remaining 3 tablespoons graham cracker crumbs in shallow dish; roll balls in crumbs to coat. Cover and refrigerate until ready to serve.

MAKES 8 SERVINGS

2 TRUFFLES PER SERVING:

calories 120

total fat 3g

saturated fat 1g

sodium 40mg

carbs 23g

fiber 1g

sugar 14g

protein 2g

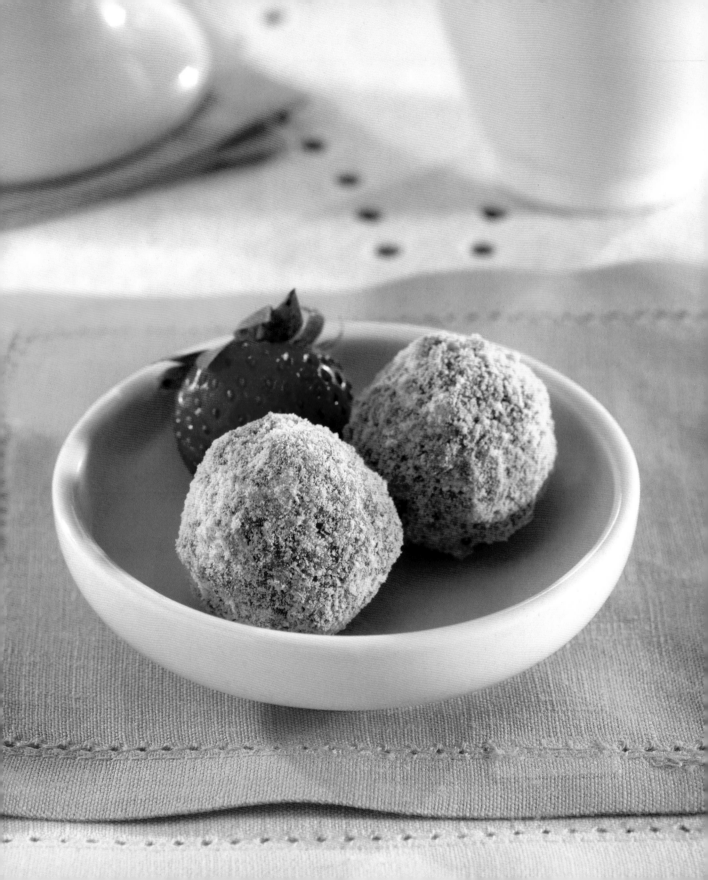

Texas Caviar

1 tablespoon vegetable oil

1 cup fresh corn (from 2 to 3 ears)

2 cans (about 15 ounces each) black-eyed peas, rinsed and drained

1 can (about 15 ounces) black beans, rinsed and drained

1 cup halved grape tomatoes

1 bell pepper (red, orange, yellow or green), finely chopped

½ cup finely chopped red onion

1 jalapeño pepper, seeded and minced

2 green onions, minced

¼ cup chopped fresh cilantro

2 tablespoons red wine vinegar

1 tablespoon plus 1 teaspoon lime juice, divided

1 teaspoon salt

1 teaspoon sugar

½ teaspoon ground cumin

½ teaspoon dried oregano

2 cloves garlic, minced

¼ cup olive oil

1 Heat vegetable oil in large skillet over high heat. Add corn; cook and stir about 3 minutes or until corn is beginning to brown in spots. Place in large bowl. Add beans, tomatoes, bell peppers, red onion, jalapeño, green onions and cilantro.

2 Combine vinegar, 1 tablespoon lime juice, 1 teaspoon salt, sugar, cumin, oregano and garlic in small bowl. Whisk in olive oil in thin, steady stream until well blended. Pour over vegetables; stir to coat.

3 Refrigerate at least 2 hours or overnight. Just before serving, stir in remaining 1 teaspoon lime juice. Taste and season with additional salt, if desired.

NOTE: Serve Texas Caviar as a dip for a crowd with corn chips or tortilla chips. It also makes a great packable lunch or side dish with tacos or grilled chicken.

MAKES ABOUT 9 CUPS (36 SERVINGS)

¼ CUP PER SERVING:

calories 50

total fat 2g

saturated fat 0g

sodium 110mg

carbs 6g

fiber 1g

sugar 1g

protein 2g

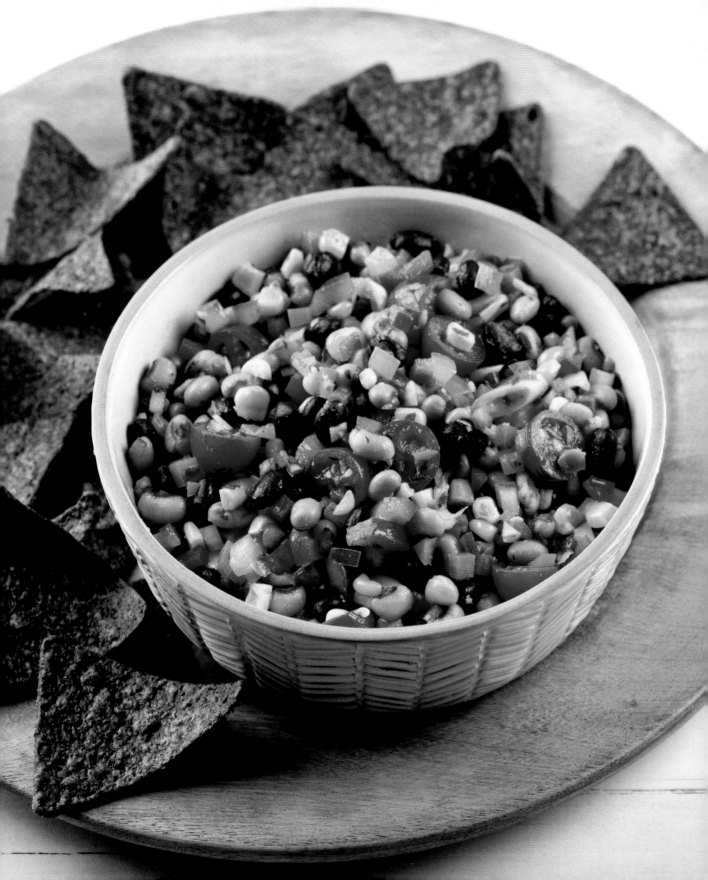

Classic Deviled Eggs

6 **eggs**

3 **tablespoons mayonnaise**

½ **teaspoon apple cider vinegar**

½ **teaspoon yellow mustard**

⅛ **teaspoon salt**

Optional toppings: black pepper, paprika, minced fresh chives and/ or minced red onion (optional)

1 Bring medium saucepan of water to a boil. Gently add eggs with slotted spoon. Reduce heat to maintain a simmer; cook 12 minutes. Meanwhile, fill medium bowl with cold water and ice cubes. Drain eggs and place in ice water; cool 10 minutes.

2 Carefully peel eggs. Cut eggs in half; place yolks in small bowl. Add mayonnaise, vinegar, mustard and salt; mash until well blended. Spoon mixture into egg whites; garnish with desired toppings.

MAKES 12 DEVILED EGGS

1 DEVILED EGG PER SERVING:

calories 30

total fat 3g

saturated fat 0g

sodium 70mg

carbs 0g

fiber 0g

sugar 0g

protein 2g

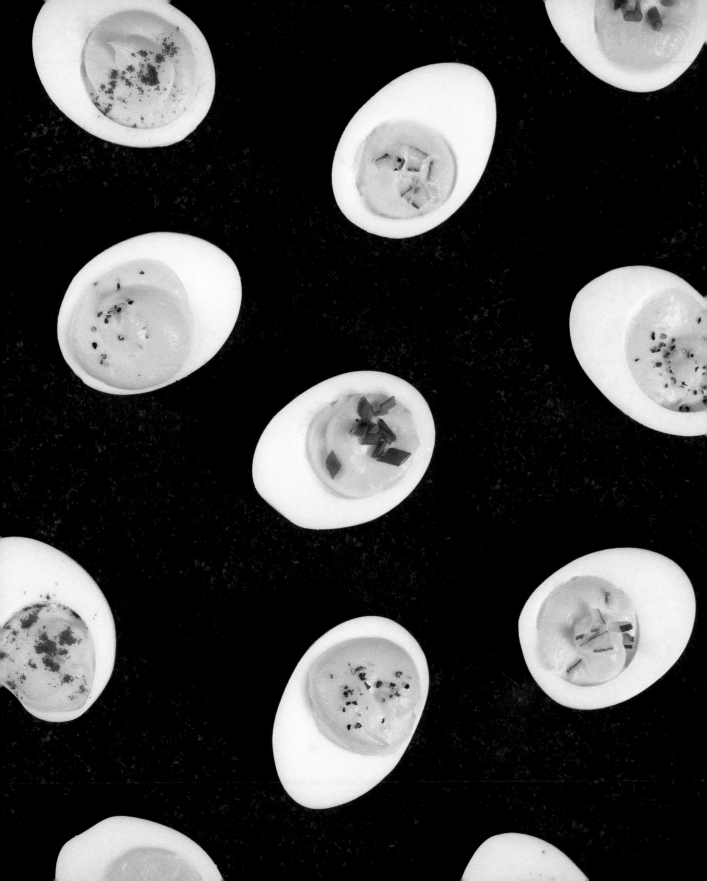

Jalapeño Poppers

10 to 12 fresh jalapeño peppers*

1 package (8 ounces) cream cheese, softened

1½ cups (6 ounces) shredded Cheddar cheese, divided

2 green onions, finely chopped

½ teaspoon onion powder

¼ teaspoon salt

⅛ teaspoon garlic powder

6 slices bacon, crisp-cooked and finely chopped

2 tablespoons almond flour or panko (optional)

2 tablespoons grated Parmesan or Romano cheese

For large jalapeño peppers, use 10. For small peppers, use 12.

1 Preheat oven to 375°F. Line baking sheet with parchment paper or foil.

2 Cut each jalapeño in half lengthwise; remove ribs and seeds.

3 Beat cream cheese, 1 cup Cheddar, green onions, onion powder, salt and garlic powder in medium bowl until well blended. Stir in bacon.

4 Fill each jalapeño half with about 1 tablespoon cheese mixture. Place on prepared baking sheet. Sprinkle with remaining ½ cup Cheddar, almond flour, if desired, and Parmesan.

5 Bake 10 to 12 minutes or until cheeses are melted and jalapeños are slightly softened.

MAKES 20 TO 24 POPPERS

1 POPPER PER SERVING:

calories 110
total fat 10g
saturated fat 5g
sodium 200mg
carbs 2g
fiber 0g
sugar 1g
protein 4g

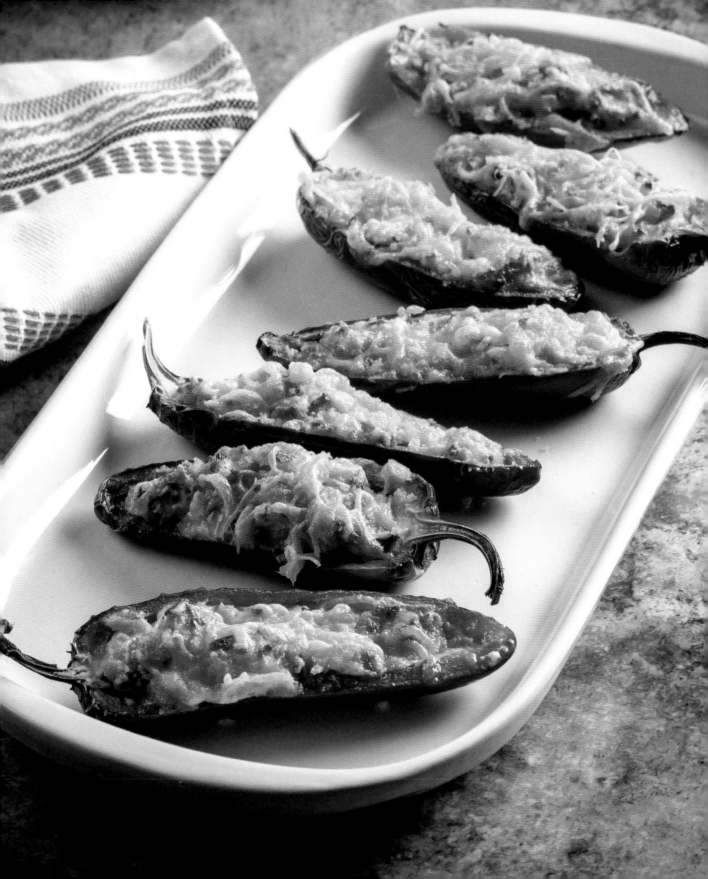

BLT Lettuce Wraps

¼ **cup plus**
   2 tablespoons
   reduced-fat
   mayonnaise

¼ **cup fat-free (skim)**
   milk

2 **teaspoons cider**
   vinegar

¼ **teaspoon garlic**
   powder

4 **cups halved grape**
   tomatoes

1 **package (16 ounces)**
   bacon, crisp-
   cooked and
   chopped

1 **cup small croutons**

8 **small butter lettuce**
   leaves

1 For dressing, whisk mayonnaise, milk, vinegar and garlic powder in small bowl until smooth and well blended.

2 Arrange tomatoes, bacon and croutons evenly on lettuce leaves. Drizzle with dressing. Serve immediately.

**MAKES
8 SERVINGS**

**1 WRAP
PER SERVING:**

calories 112
total fat 7g
saturated
   fat 2g
sodium
   388mg
carbs 8g
fiber 1g
sugar 3g
protein 6g

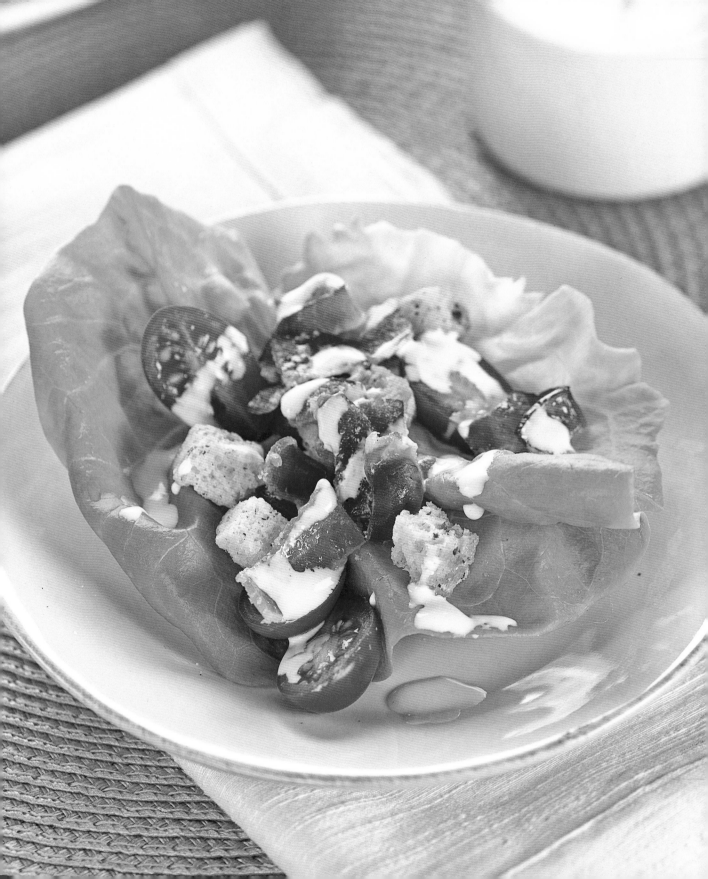

Mojito Shrimp Cocktail

1 **pound frozen medium raw shrimp, deveined but not peeled (with tails on)**

1 **cup plus 2 tablespoons prepared mojito cocktail mix, divided**

2 **tablespoons olive oil**

1 **jar (12 ounces) shrimp cocktail sauce**

1 Place shrimp in large shallow glass dish. Pour 1 cup mojito mix over shrimp to cover. (Separate shrimp as much as possible to aid thawing.) Marinate in refrigerator 10 to 24 hours or until thawed, stirring shrimp once or twice.

2 Prepare grill for direct cooking. Drain shrimp; discard marinade. *Do not peel.* Pat dry and place in large bowl. Drizzle with oil; toss to coat.

3 Grill shrimp over medium-high heat on grill topper* 10 to 15 minutes or until shrimp are pink and opaque, turning once. Refrigerate until ready to serve.

4 Pour cocktail sauce into serving bowl; add remaining 1 to 2 tablespoons mojito mix and stir to combine. Serve with shrimp.

Shrimp may also be cooked in a grill pan.

MAKES 8 SERVINGS

$\frac{1}{8}$ OF TOTAL RECIPE PER SERVING:

calories 130
total fat 4g
saturated fat 1g
sodium 820mg
carbs 12g
fiber 1g
sugar 8g
protein 8g

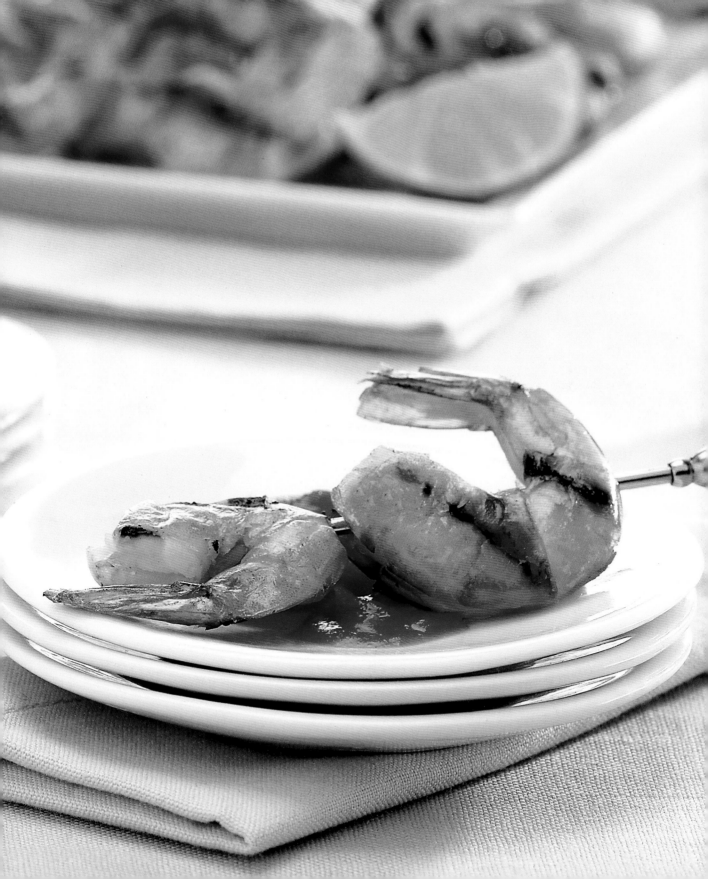

INDEX

INDEX

Metric Conversion Chart

VOLUME MEASUREMENTS (dry)

⅛ teaspoon = 0.5 mL
¼ teaspoon = 1 mL
½ teaspoon = 2 mL
¾ teaspoon = 4 mL
1 teaspoon = 5 mL
1 tablespoon = 15 mL
2 tablespoons = 30 mL
¼ cup = 60 mL
⅓ cup = 75 mL
½ cup = 125 mL
⅔ cup = 150 mL
¾ cup = 175 mL
1 cup = 250 mL
2 cups = 1 pint = 500 mL
3 cups = 750 mL
4 cups = 1 quart = 1 L

VOLUME MEASUREMENTS (fluid)

1 fluid ounce (2 tablespoons) = 30 mL
4 fluid ounces (½ cup) = 125 mL
8 fluid ounces (1 cup) = 250 mL
12 fluid ounces (1½ cups) = 375 mL
16 fluid ounces (2 cups) = 500 mL

WEIGHTS (mass)

½ ounce = 15 g
1 ounce = 30 g
3 ounces = 90 g
4 ounces = 120 g
8 ounces = 225 g
10 ounces = 285 g
12 ounces = 360 g
16 ounces = 1 pound = 450 g

DIMENSIONS

1/16 inch = 2 mm
⅛ inch = 3 mm
¼ inch = 6 mm
½ inch = 1.5 cm
¾ inch = 2 cm
1 inch = 2.5 cm

OVEN TEMPERATURES

250°F = 120°C
275°F = 140°C
300°F = 150°C
325°F = 160°C
350°F = 180°C
375°F = 190°C
400°F = 200°C
425°F = 220°C
450°F = 230°C

BAKING PAN SIZES

Utensil	Size in Inches/Quarts	Metric Volume	Size in Centimeters
Baking or Cake Pan (square or rectangular)	8×8×2	2 L	20×20×5
	9×9×2	2.5 L	23×23×5
	12×8×2	3 L	30×20×5
	13×9×2	3.5 L	33×23×5
Loaf Pan	8×4×3	1.5 L	20×10×7
	9×5×3	2 L	23×13×7
Round Layer Cake Pan	8×1½	1.2 L	20×4
	9×1½	1.5 L	23×4
Pie Plate	8×1¼	750 mL	20×3
	9×1¼	1 L	23×3
Baking Dish or Casserole	1 quart	1 L	—
	1½ quart	1.5 L	—
	2 quart	2 L	—